Seek
Discover
Transform

A Path to Creating a Purpose-Filled Life

LAURA MACDONELL

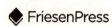 FriesenPress

One Printers Way
Altona, MB R0G 0B0
Canada

www.friesenpress.com

ISBN
978-1-03-917570-9 (Hardcover)
978-1-03-917569-3 (Paperback)
978-1-03-917571-6 (eBook)

Self-Help, Motivational & Inspirational

Distributed to the trade by The Ingram Book Company

This book is dedicated to my children Sidney and Logan, who inspire me to live my life with purpose and love. May you both seek your true calling, discover what brings you joy and create a purpose-filled life!

TABLE OF CONTENTS

INTRODUCTION

I struggled with how to begin this book. What began as an outpouring of my soul reflected as words on a page, slowly transformed into a structured book. As my own healing journey unfolded in the duration of writing this book, I decided to tune into my own inner wisdom and trust my intuition on what to include and what not to include. I took parts out, then I was guided to put them back in. It may not have been the traditionally perceived "right" way to write a book, but it was the heartfelt way. In doing so, I believe and hope I'm able to connect with you from a more authentic space. It may not be perfect, but it is real.

So, I begin with my truth and my lived experiences, with the hope that you, the reader, will be inspired to connect deeper with your truest, most authentic SELF, discover your purpose, and share your gifts generously with your community. Perhaps you will begin a new journey, dust off a forgotten project, or live more fully on the path you are on. Above all, my intention is to guide you to not only listen to the quiet whispers of your soul but to support you into taking inspired action, bringing your dreams into reality.

The answer you've been searching for—your life's purpose, is right here—buried under fear, doubt, and limiting beliefs. The exercises and reflection questions in each chapter will support you in recognizing and working with these beliefs so that you can begin to create a purpose-driven life of true freedom. Your experiences will not always be roses and sunshine, but by following the callings of your innermost, truest self you will experience deep fulfillment.

BEGINNINGS

When I was fourteen, I picked up my first personal development book called *The Nature of Change*. It was to be the first of many. I have never been a fan of change and was struggling with the news that our family was moving to a new city. Shortly after, I found a book called *You Are Physic*. I thought, if I couldn't control my external circumstances, then I better be able to predict them so I could at least be prepared.

I continued to pursue personal growth and development into my teenage years and adult life. My curious mind was always full of deep questions: Why am I here? What's my purpose? What will make me happy? What's the point of this life? Although many others have contemplated these types of questions, for me, it led to feeling anxious and worried that I didn't know my life's purpose. What if I was living someone else's version of my life?

When I was twenty-three years old, I purchased the family business from my parents. For twenty-two years, I managed and operated the company, and I loved many parts of it—mainly that it was in the health and well-being sector, an area I'm still very passionate about. Being self-employed also allowed me many freedoms I would not have had otherwise. I truly feel humbly blessed for the opportunity I had at such a young age.

But even though I was outwardly successful, I felt restless, like there was something more I was meant to do—my true calling. I continued to read dozens of self-help books, but none of them really propelled me to take aligned action. I learned a lot, and for that, I'm extremely grateful. What I felt was missing from many of the books I'd read, were specific actions I could take each day that would get me one step closer to not only discovering but living a life that brought me true fulfillment and joy.

In 2013, I lost my dad suddenly to pancreatic cancer. He was only sixty-six and had a real zest for life right up until he died.

Everything changed for me after his death. I lost my own zest for life and began just going through the motions day after day. I was in deep grief but didn't realize the full extent of it at the time. But it was from this dark place that a tiny spark began to flicker.

At the time, I had been practising yoga regularly for about fifteen years and I was very passionate about it. After the death of my dad, I dove in even deeper, seeking solace from the heaviness I felt. Up until then I was mainly interested in the physical benefits of yoga. Little did I know what was possible when I began to study this ancient practice. In 2016, I had the opportunity to attend a yoga teacher training program and took it. Shortly after that I became a meditation facilitator. I taught yoga classes, assisted in leading yoga teacher trainings and foundational yoga courses as well as life design workshops. My training continued into 2019 achieving five hundred hours of yoga teacher training.

The self-inquiry work that follows in this book is a compilation of what I've learned in my trainings and the many spiritual texts I've studied by leading scientists, yogis, and gurus. Bringing these teachings together, I developed a six-step process for discovering, creating, and living your life's purpose. It is action-based, but simple and easy to do at your own pace.

This process propelled me out of anxiety, confusion, and lack of confidence. For so many years I struggled to find my purpose and I questioned my contribution to society. In this book we'll examine the practical tools and insights that helped me move from confusion and self-doubt to clarity and confidence. I will guide you to uncover your truest self, discover your purpose and create a life you love.

You will:

- Become aware of how the voice in your head creates your feelings, beliefs, actions and, ultimately, your life.
- Learn the five disguises of fear and how these hidden fears block the path to living your most fulfilling life.

- Learn why certain patterns in your life continue to repeat over and over again and how to create new patterns.
- Learn valuable tools that will bring you back to your true self when you get pulled off course.
- Learn how to use the six-step recipe for creating your most fulfilling life.
- Learn how to make these new habits stick to create changes long after you've completed this book.
- Learn how your greater self-awareness affects the global community.

The book is divided into three parts. Each part is important to creating the blueprint of your desired path. At the end of each chapter there are reflection questions that help you gain insight and clarity. There are also practices within the chapters to help you stay on track.

Part 1—SEEK: This part begins by uncovering the layers of beliefs you have about yourself that limit you from reaching your greatest potential. Through upbringing, cultural constructs, and programming, you have formed these beliefs not only about yourself, but about the world you live in. Some may be valuable, but others keep you constrained.

Part 2—DISCOVER: Once you've excavated and reflected on the hidden parts of your sub-conscious mind and practised the exercises in Part 1, you will now dive further into identifying your core values, passions, strengths, skills, and goals. This is where you will learn the six-step process for creating a life of fulfillment and purpose. With further reflection questions and exercises, you will be guided into a deeper sense of clarity and self-awareness that will set you up for Part 3.

Part 3—TRANSFORM: The last section is about how to take action in your daily life and remain accountable so you can experience tangible results. Through movement and managing the day-to-day emotions and stress of daily life, you will learn how to stay focused even amidst challenges and setbacks.

It is up to you now to not only read the words on the pages but choose to embody the suggestions and answer the reflection questions, so you can begin the create your very best life. The power is within you!

"You are the dreamer of your dream that is your life."
Gabrielle Bernstein

PART 1: SEEK

Your thoughts and beliefs create your behaviours.
Your behaviours create your actions.
Your actions create your life.

CHAPTER 1

WAKING UP

GREMLINS

It was the summer of 2016, as I sat surrounded by fifty other keen yogis at a retreat centre in Northern Ontario, eager with pen and notebook, to learn how to become a yoga teacher. It would be a two-week intensive training with very little time off. I thought I knew what I was getting myself into, but what I learned was far beyond what I could have imagined.

The training was intense for me—physically, mentally, and emotionally. I thought I'd show up, learn the poses, teach the class. How hard could it be? I'd been practising as a student for fifteen years so I should already know most of this stuff already. I admit, I was naïve to the ancient teachings. In our Western culture, yoga has been diminished to a series of postures to improve flexibility and mobility. Although this is a large part of yoga, I was about to learn what really excited me about the practice—the self-inquiry and expansion of self-awareness.

One particular part of the training that really stuck for me was the Gremlins session. You may remember the 1980s movie *Gremlins*. It's about these cute little cuddly creatures that, when given food after midnight, turn into mean, ugly, disturbing creatures that wreak havoc on everything they come in contact with. The Gremlins, in this training, illustrated how your thoughts can become like gremlins. They can take you down a rabbit hole of darkness with unkind words, discouragement, doubt, and fear. You have so many great beautiful thoughts, great ideas, passions, goals—you are a good person. You have a path you are meant to walk down. Then there are the gremlins.

The gremlins show up when we get scared. They are the thoughts that say, "Who are you to write that book, lead that class, open that business, paint those pictures, travel the world, move to the islands, or quit the job that you hate? Do you really think you have enough time, money, support, ambition? So many people are already doing what you want to do. So many people have failed, you'll see. You're not talented enough, strong enough, motivated enough. It will never work. Scratch that idea. Back to work, back to the comfort of what you know. It's safe there. You're protected. You won't get hurt if you stay where you are. Your life is good, it's fine. Just be grateful for what you have and let your dream settle back down." Sound familiar?

That is a gremlin. That is the worst kind of friend to have, and yet it's in there, always conversing with you, even when you aren't fully aware of it. In fact, our thoughts often aren't even in our conscious awareness. They happen in our subconscious mind so quickly that we don't have a chance to interrupt them. The gremlins are there in the biggest dreams of your life and in your everyday interactions. "Don't say that. You might sound stupid. Don't speak up. Your boss will get upset with you. You'll feel so embarrassed. Quiet, safe, this moment will pass, yes, safe."

When this type of negative thinking becomes habitual, it may seem like nothing works out for you. You may fall into complaint mode all the time and once you land in victimhood it can sometimes feel challenging to pull yourself out. It feels heavy and is disempowering when you're stuck in this downward spiral.

Imagine now that your best friend or your child has come to you, and they are stuck in this pattern of negative thinking. How would you speak to them? What words of encouragement would you say to them? How would you support them?

Once you become aware of the voice in your head, you'll start to notice all the ways you put yourself down or talk yourself out of reaching towards a goal or dream. Within this spark of awareness is the opportunity to befriend your gremlins and speak to them the way you would a loved one. With some practise, you'll begin to rewrite the negative script with a more supportive one. At the end of the chapter is an exercise to assist you in becoming aware and moving beyond habitual thoughts patterns.

THE VOICE IN YOUR HEAD

What is this voice in your head that directs your life? Where did the gremlins come from? Most importantly, how can you quiet them when they show up so loudly?

What Is The Voice in Your Head?

Many philosophers and spiritual leaders have spent countless hours and written thousands of books on who or what it is that is speaking to us in our thoughts every day. The quest for the origin of this voice continues. My best explanation is that this voice— sometimes called the ego—is a learned voice that is part of our smaller SELF. Spiritualist teacher Don Miguel Ruiz puts it this way in *The Voice of Knowledge: A Practical Guide to Inner Peace*: "The voice in our head comes after we learn language, then different points of view, then all the judgement and lies" (p. 11). Our true SELF or our higher SELF is the observer of this voice.

Where Did the Voice Come From?

The voice is learned from everything we have ever heard, read, and observed. In his research, cell biologist and author of *Biology of Belief,* Bruce Lipton explores how from birth until age seven our brains are primarily in a theta vibration, or hypnosis state. In this state, we are like sponges, absorbing our environment without consciously choosing to. Every thought we've had from the moment we began to understand and speak our language becomes the "voice in our head." But does this voice speak the truth, or does it tell you lies? Is it supporting your growth, or isn't it? To answer these questions, you must become attentive enough to hear the voice and ultimately silence it long enough to have the opportunity to decide.

How Can the Voice Be Quieted?

The first step is awareness. Once you begin to notice the voice you are in a more powerful position because you now have a choice, to believe the voice or not. Most of the time we're just out there running on autopilot. Our thoughts and beliefs create patterns in our brains. In an effort to exert the least amount of energy and free up space to take in external stimuli, the brain turns the thought pattern into a habit. *Science Connected Magazine* explains how habits are formed: "Our brains form neural pathways—connections between neurons—that get stronger the more often we perform a task. And when we perform a task enough times, we no longer have to think about how it's done. This is when it becomes a habit."

This is often a good thing. If you have been driving a car for some time, you no longer have to consciously think about which pedal is the gas and which one is the brake. If you drive the same route to work each day, you may arrive and wonder how you got there. You no longer have to get out the GPS and find your way there. Habits are important. Yet, thought patterns or habits that do not serve you in a positive way also run on autopilot, and thereby create your behaviours and your actions that in turn create your life unconsciously. Further, the stronger you feel about an event in your life, the stronger are the neural pathway connections that form. The good news is that you can retrain your brain. As with learning a new skill, it takes time to unlearn old ways of being, but it is possible.

CHALLENGING YOUR THOUGHTS

"Anxious, fearful thoughts are not telling us the truth, they are only making us afraid."

—Deepak Chopra

We have over 40,000 thoughts a day. Is it possible to be aware of all of them? Likely not. There are some, however, that stick. And what I mean by "stick" is they take you into a story. I'm speaking specifically here about the negative thought patterns that share the following characteristics:

1. They're repetitive: when you get triggered by a situation or fear, a thought spiral begins that feels very familiar.

2. They're easy to justify: you can conjure up physical evidence proving they're right.

3. They're not very supportive and often seek to find the worst-case scenario.

4. They stir up emotions of fear, anger, envy, or sadness.

5. They're a reflection of the past—of unhealed wounds.

6. They are NOT true.

Negative automatic thoughts happen so quickly, like lightning strikes, and the more they strike, the more powerful they become until they have created damage. Unless you become aware of this thought and ask yourself, "Is it true?", it will be very difficult to disengage from its power.

You can take this awareness one step further:

1. Notice the negative thought.

2. Ask, "Is it true?"

3. Replace it with a thought that creates a more desirable outcome.

4. Use this new positive thought as your mantra (a statement that's repeated frequently) whenever the "gremlin" arrives.

5. Better still, use this mantra when things are going well-look for evidence to support the new thought.

Consider the results of replacing just one negative thought pattern with a more supportive statement. From this new point of awareness, you will begin to see evidence around you affirming the supportive thought. You will move from a place of disempowerment into conscious creation. Practice and patience with yourself are important. When you begin to intentionally step into your personal growth, the world will provide you with many opportunities to practice your new skill. They may not always be enjoyable, but this practice is necessary if you want to experience real changes in your life.

I recently took time off work and off writing. It was a great time to recharge and remember what things really make me feel fulfilled and energized. Every day I walked, meditated, did yoga, and played board games with my kids and husband. I caught up with family and friends who live far away and had some really nice conversations. Fast forward to day one back to work and writing, and some gremlins started to re-emerge. Before, I would not have noticed these gremlins, but this time something caught my attention.

As I recommitted to my writing, the instant, automatic response came that if I focus just an hour and a half a day on writing my book, then my other business will go downhill. I won't have the time and energy to devote to my other business and therefore it will fail. Whoa, is that true? Is that what I've been telling myself numerous times a day? Is that the statement that's creating my reality? The truth is, my other business won't fail if I devote some time to writing each day.

What if my thought changed to, "When I spend an hour and a half writing every day, I am more effective and creative at work." I'm happier, more aware, and taking time for myself means I give my team more autonomy and freedom to do their work, so they also benefit. This sounds more supportive of the reality I actually want to create.

How can you apply this to your own life? What can you tell yourself instead when a negative thought pattern comes up?

This is a daily moment-by-moment practice. Your life will give you multiple opportunities a day to witness these types of thoughts. It's up to you to either choose to believe them or use them to propel yourself forward by choosing thoughts that strengthen you.

MEDITATION

The practice of meditation is a great tool that can assist you in becoming more aware of your thoughts. Meditation has been used by cultures around the world for thousands of years. It's a practice used to focus the mind and create a heightened state of awareness. There are many scientifically proven benefits of meditation as well, including stress reduction, blood pressure regulation, improved sleep, reduced anxiety, immune support, headache relief, and enhanced self-awareness.

If you're new to meditation, it may be uncomfortable and challenging to quiet the inner voice. You may want to move. You will likely experience many thoughts. The default of continually thinking is strong, but just like building stronger muscles in the body, it takes consistency and practice. You may begin noticing how every day your thoughts can be so different—quiet one day, loud and distracting the next. What's really powerful, though, is when you start to become aware of repetitive thoughts and beliefs. It's from this point that you can begin to choose new thoughts and create the reality you desire.

There are so many apps and online options to choose from that offer guided meditations. It's great to try out a few and see what fits with you. I personally love the Deepak Chopra app. It has many options, from three minutes up to twenty minutes with new meditations added daily.

Here is an example of meditation in practice: find a quiet comfortable seat where you won't be interrupted. Close your eyes and put your attention on your breath coming in and out through your nose. Relax your shoulders and sit up tall. Simply begin to notice your thoughts. Pay attention to how you feel right then in that moment. There is no right or wrong. Trust what comes up; trust the knowing deep within you. Thoughts will flow in and out. I like to imagine them as clouds floating by in the blue sky. You may get attached to a thought—become aware of it then let it go. When you get distracted by the racing mind, put your attention back on your breath flowing in and out of your nostrils. Don't worry if your mind wanders the entire time. Just sit and observe without judgment for a few minutes. If you can quiet the mind long enough, you get a chance to listen deeply.

It took me an entire year of regular meditation practice to really begin to enjoy meditating. With on again off again commitment, meditation has literally saved me from so much anxiety and racing thoughts. It also helped me focus on what I truly wanted in my life. So don't give up on it. Keep coming back when you fall off track.

If you feel uncertain about meditating, I get it. It's not always easy to sit still in silence. Look at it this way; you don't have to meditate, you simply have to sit quietly for a few minutes a day to tune into your breath, in and out. Think of it as a positive timeout for grownups.

REFLECTION

1. Identify a common negative thought pattern that you believe to be true about yourself and your life?

2. If that thought pattern was absolutely without a doubt NOT TRUE, what positive thought could you replace it with?

3. How could this new, more supportive thought impact your decisions?

4. Action step: try a five-minute meditation every morning for the next seven days. Notice how this habit affects your physical, mental, and emotional states.

"Everything you want is on the other side of fear."

— Jack Canfield

CHAPTER 2

THE FIVE DISGUISES OF FEAR

Fear is primal. Our knee-jerk reaction when facing danger is to run to safety, stay and fight, or freeze. When danger arises, it threatens our survival, so we choose quickly in the moment what to do. But what about the not-so-obvious part of fear that has become a part of our unconscious reactions? Fear can be sneaky and hide behind some clever everyday disguises. I've identified five ways in which the mind seeks to protect us and hide us from the fears that lie just beneath the surface.

THE FIVE DISGUISES OF FEAR

1. Guilt

2. People pleasing

3. Procrastination

4. Overachieving

5. Control

DISGUISE #1: GUILT

Let's start off with this very common feeling—guilt. Guilt is like a ping-pong game between our own desire and what we believe we should be doing or should have done. The "shoulds" that stick are different for everyone, depending on culture, age, gender, upbringing, and socioeconomic status. There also many "shoulds" that we share with the collective. As a mother, I experience guilt. The moment I want to go to yoga class or sit and read a book, someone needs something from me. The puppy dog eyes come out, or I hear the "you're going to yoga again" comment. Ugh . . . the guilt. I *should* be here 24/7 for my kids; after all, I birthed them into the world. So, the entire time I'm taking a yoga class or reading a book, the self-care turns into negative, guilty self-talk. This is completely normal: most parents feel the need to prioritize their children's needs over their own.

Similar "should" feelings can also arise in a work situation. You should be staying late to finish that report. You should be answering emails from home like all your other colleagues are doing.

Consider how guilt is fear in disguise. If you look below the surface of guilt, you'll find the deeper beliefs, which may be fear of:

- not being good enough
- not being accepted
- being undervalued
- missing an opportunity
- being judged poorly

If one of these beliefs is subconsciously running the show, your reaction may be to say yes and agree to do something that you really wanted to say no to. Guilt can also lead you to compromise taking care of your own needs in favour of satisfying someone else's.

Start to pay attention to the daily choices you make and how they make you feel. Have certain tasks just become a chore that you've chosen to do out of guilt or habit? Or are you performing your tasks with joy and creation? Awareness starts with noticing the day-to-day seemingly routine tasks and expands out to the bigger choices in your life.

Similar threads of thoughts weave in and out of many other bigger situations. These thoughts are indicator lights that you can use to bring greater awareness to subconscious fear-based belief patterns. Guilt may be the surface level experience, but looking deeper, ask yourself: why do you feel guilty?

Is there something you continue to do out of guilt? What fear could that feeling of guilt be covering up?

Taking this further, does this fear block you from doing what you really want to do or expressing yourself in a creative way— from building your own business to creating your artwork or sharing your ideas on a project at work?

When I started my regular yoga practice, I felt a tremendous amount of guilt for starting work a bit later one day a week. The narrative that ran through my head while I was trying to be Zen and do yoga was, "What will happen if I'm not there? What will my staff think of me? Am I setting a good example? A boss is supposed to lead by example, so I need to be available to prove this is how you work hard." The buried fear was that I would be judged as a poor leader, that I was not good enough.

At the time, I was reading *The Art of Extreme Self-Care* by Cheryl Richardson, and I read something profound that really stuck with me. Instead of feeling guilty for taking care of myself, I could change the narrative to, "The more I take care of myself, the more my business will flourish." So, every time I felt guilty, I would repeat this mantra during yoga class. By doing this I was able to flip the script and begin to create a new reality for myself.

Beginning to pay attention is the first step. Without awareness of the narrative, you won't be able to take action and create the change you desire, even if it's simply enjoying a more "Zen" yoga class.

REFLECTION

1. What are some common things you tell yourself when you feel passionate about a step forward in your life but then back out?

2. What do your inner gremlins say to you when you need to do something for yourself--like leave work early for dinner with your family, or your child's soccer game, or when you want to try a new exercise class or learn to paint?

3. What can you say instead to flip the script and begin to create a more supportive environment for your goals to flourish in?

DISGUISE #2: PEOPLE PLEASING

People-pleasing is rooted in the fear that you will not be accepted for being your authentic self.

The Innate Need to Conform

As humans, we have an innate need to fit in and be liked and accepted by our peers. Evolution shows us that those who fit into the tribe have a better chance of survival than those who are outcast and banished from their communities. In *A Learning Mind* blog post, Ruth Newton, MA, BA, explains the survival value of conformity:

Conformity appeared when our ancestors were trying to survive through getting together and forming tribes. In those wild dangerous times, it was impossible to survive on one's own, so early humans aligned with a group in order to get food and protection from the numerous threats. Even if one person would probably be able to find some food to survive, they couldn't fight on their own against the countless predators that attacked them. No need to say that fighting off these attacks as a group was much more effective, which ensured humans' survival. Thus, the primary aim of conformity was the survival of our species.

Fitting in at its most primal level satisfies our need for survival. But, by absently conforming to the social structure without taking the time to think critically, you are doing a disservice to yourself and to society at large. Conformity can hold you back from exploring and expressing your true self.

Fitting in at the expense of your own well-being moves you into the phase of active people pleasing. Active people pleasing is a full-time job. It's exhausting and it never ends because it is literally impossible to manage the behaviours of other people. It is a losing battle and yet fear of being ousted from the tribe can keep you stuck in this continual cycle. The harm of staying in this cycle is resentment, exhaustion, and not tending to your own wants, needs, and dreams.

Conditioning

The impulse to want to please others, fit in, and be accepted varies with each person, and is part of our conditioning and upbringing. The conditioning begins at home, and then solidifies when we go to school.

With practice, we can get really good at hiding our true selves in order to fit in. I grew up with three siblings, smack dab in the middle, child number three. In larger families, it's easy to hide. I grew up in a culture that praised children who were quiet, well-behaved, and followed the rules. This may be true for you, too.

Think back to when you were at school. As children, we are trained to sit still, be quiet, and listen to the teacher. Instilling this respect for others is important. Rules are made to keep order, yet they can become very constraining, especially for many children who have an innate curiosity for learning and the energy to move. The ones who don't follow or who question the rules are sent away to the principal's office for punishment or, even worse, reprimanded and shamed in front of the entire class. The "good kids," the ones who follow the rules, don't get in trouble, and are therefore rewarded. It's no wonder so many of us begin to fit ourselves into this box of good behaviour. It's easier to fit in than to rebel. Those who rebel or challenge the rules have more difficulty functioning in society.

My mom often tells me how I would punish myself, as early as age three, to avoid being disciplined by her and my dad. It's pretty ingenious for a three-year-old to punish herself instead of letting others control the consequence. But as an adult, that form of self-punishment can get worse—running a mile to "work off" one cookie or punishing yourself with negative self-talk for not getting a "good enough" grade at school. And it can also push you into the people-pleasing cycle.

For example, our culture reveres women for being thin and young. Many women and girls go to great lengths to fit this ideal at the expense of their health. I cannot say I haven't fallen victim to this pressure. I exercised quite a bit when I was younger to maintain a certain body weight and be accepted. If I ate a big meal or dessert, I felt pressure to work it off, so exercise became a form of punishment. You likely have your own version of negative self-talk.

Ask yourself, who are you trying to please? Your peers, parents, boss, colleagues, strangers, society at large? Perhaps you're so hard on yourself because you believe this is what everyone wants from you. Is this people-pleasing behaviour coming at the expense of your well-being? And is it what you really want? Does it make you feel good? What fears are present when you feel the need to over-please at the expense of your own well-being?

Breaking the People-Pleasing Cycle

Breaking free of the people-pleasing cycle may feel selfish at the start but taking care of yourself doesn't mean you start to ignore everyone else around you. It doesn't mean you stop helping others. It doesn't mean you don't care. It means you begin showing up authentically and lovingly for others as well as for yourself.

Setting boundaries is the most impactful step you can take to start breaking free of this pattern. Boundaries are also an act of self-love.

There are three types of boundaries:

1. Physical

2. Emotional

3. Spiritual

I'm not great at setting boundaries, so I have to work at it every day. The downside of not setting boundaries, in addition to creating resentment, is that situations continue to occur that really bother you. You effectively teach others how to treat you—and that it's okay to behave a certain way around you. By setting clear boundaries, you can communicate what is and isn't acceptable to you in any given situation.

Physical boundaries

Physical boundaries are the more tangible things you need to be your best self. For example, I need fresh air, nature, exercise, yoga, and a good sweaty workout once in a while to feel physically good. My body needs to move, stretch, and breathe deeply to clear out stuck energy and ensure I will be healthy and nimble for many years to come. I also need quiet to think, to write and to do my best work. Some people like background sounds or music or constant feedback from others. For me, that's a distraction and takes me out of what I need to focus on. I have to set physical boundaries or else I don't get much quality work done, or I feel physically sore or in pain, and become moody.

With awareness, you will begin to know what you physically need to function optimally. What type of environment do you function best in? When does your body feel most at ease? When do you feel most energized? For me, sometimes even indoor lighting can be physically draining. Lighting in big-box stores can be so harsh that it completely drains my energy in a short amount of time.

Begin to notice when you feel drained. Once you have this awareness, you can start to set some physical boundaries that work for you instead of against you. Communicate these preferences to those who you interact with. Protecting your physical space and needs will provide you with more energy to do your job, interact with your kids, your friends, and your family. When the physical space feels good, you will feel good.

Emotional boundaries

Your emotional body is active all day long, just as your physical body is. It just may be more subtle, so you may not even notice it. Emotions are like waves: they move in and out fluidly throughout the day. Some emotions may hold on a little longer but eventually they pass. Starting the day with one simple question will help you to become aware of what emotion may be driving your day. How do I feel today?

The answer will help you to identify what emotions may be driving your conversations, decisions, and reactions. It will also help you to see what support you may need and what type of activities to engage in. Most importantly, this awareness allows you to set your emotions apart from others. An emotional boundary is a clear line of what is and what is not yours to deal with.

Have you ever been energetic, happy, and excited to start your day, but then meet someone who emotionally dumps all their complaints on you? This can be a serious downer. Perhaps you feel bad for this person and genuinely want to help them, so you begin to take on their issues as your own. It may feel like you're being unsympathetic if you begin to detach from this type of interaction and set an emotional boundary. Genuine empathy, however, is the power to listen deeply without taking on the other person's pain and allowing them to find the tools to bring themselves out of their own pain. The people-pleasing part of you will want to be the saviour and fix their problems.

Setting emotional boundaries and being empathetic toward others requires creating a safety net around yourself. You need to protect and conserve your energy so you can be a source of support for others without becoming completely drained. Protect your own energy. And be aware of when you're showing up as the fixer, the pleaser.

Spiritual boundaries

Setting spiritual boundaries starts with becoming clear on your beliefs. It's like tuning into your internal moral compass and choosing each day to live by your spiritual code. Spirituality is not religion, although your religious beliefs may help form the basis for your spiritual beliefs. Wisdom traditions from around the world share many core beliefs—the most common being the belief in a Divine Source of creation. Whether you call it God, Allah, Mohammed, or Source Energy, most people believe in a creative power bigger than themselves. These traditions also share a similar moral code that includes respecting fellow humans, treating others with kindness, giving back and helping those in need, speaking truthfully, and doing no harm to others.

Spiritual boundaries allow us to deeply honour our own values. They govern the beliefs we hold and how we put them into practice. They provide a container in which to hold and practice the things that bring us closer to divinity or universal consciousness. When you are clear on your values, you build a base to lean into when you have difficult decisions to make. When you get clear on and begin to honour your beliefs, you learn to trust yourself. You know that the decisions you make are bound in your own truth. You become unshakable, steady, and strong. When the external world begins to change around you, you remain rooted in your true nature. Being grounded in your SELF also allows you to be flexible when the flow of your life changes.

Spiritual boundaries are based on truth, love, kindness, compassion, acceptance, and humility. Part of having boundaries includes respecting the beliefs of others. Just because you have a belief does not mean it is the only truth. It may be your truth, but holding space by purely listening without forcing your beliefs on others allows for deeper connections and acceptance. Move from judgment to curiosity.

REFLECTION

1. Think of a situation when you said yes but you wanted to say no. What fear was present when you made the choice? What was the result?

2. Think of a time when you said no but you wanted to say yes. What fear present was when you made the choice? What was the result?

3. List three physical, emotional, and spiritual boundaries that will help you to move out of people pleasing and into a more supportive environment for yourself.

Physical   Emotional   Spiritual

_____   _____   _____

_____   _____   _____

_____   _____   _____

Examples of physical boundaries

- Schedule time in your calendar for a workout
- Bring beauty into your home with fresh flowers or art that you love
- Keep your physical space clean and tidy
- Get rid of clutter: Clean out old clothing and trinkets that you no longer use

Examples of emotional boundaries

- Time:
  - Don't overcommit
  - Ask for help
  - Delegate when you have too much to do
- Personal:
  - Speak up if you feel your needs aren't being met
  - Value your own perspective and experience

- Don't let people lie to you, bully you or deceive you (teach others how to treat you)

Examples of spiritual boundaries

- Set time aside to develop a spiritual practice you resonate with: meditation, prayer, reflection, books
- Join a like-minded community group
- Volunteer your time for a cause you believe in
- Listen to peaceful music
- Light incense or a white candle

DISGUISE #3: OVERACHIEVING

There is nothing wrong with working hard for what you want out of life. In fact, creating a life you love requires you to commit to doing some tough work. It requires resilience when challenges are thrown at you, and it requires you to examine the self-limiting beliefs you have that are holding you back from choosing to move forward. There is nothing wrong with being externally successful in a career you love, or with the family you raise, or in a project that has deep meaning to you. But if your success is built on fear, that sense of achievement will only be momentary and fleeting. You may believe that certain achievements—having a bigger house, reaching a sales target, getting a promotion, or whatever else you consider success—will finally make you happy or make someone you care about happy. The downside of this type of success is that you enter a cycle of constant searching. It becomes your full-time job.

I've been an overachiever most of my life. Early on, it began with me wanting to impress others and be liked and accepted by my teachers and parents by doing well at school and winning awards. As I got older, this need for acceptance became ingrained even deeper. It became a habit and, ultimately, a mask. Overachieving became a way to hide my fear of failure.

In my mid-twenties, I started seeing a chiropractor. He had a unique way of looking at the whole person from an intuitive perspective. Our first appointment was a full assessment of my physical complaints, my spinal alignment, and so on. But then he asked me what my greatest fear was. Without a pause I blurted out, "My greatest fear is failure." I don't know where it came from or why this moment has stuck with me for all these years. But there it was, out in the open. Some people, myself included, believe that we hold our emotions in our bodies. We are more than just physical beings. We are emotional beings.

Years later, as I studied more about the body and physical disease, I learned that the chiropractor's question, which seemed irrelevant at the time, was a key to treating my lower back pain. Louise L. Hay's book *You Can Heal Your Life* is about how our emotions affect our physical health. By implementing Hay's recommendations, I was able to heal many of my physical ailments, from digestive issues to canker sores to anxiety.

Success on the outside meant everything was great on the inside and I had found a way to outrun failure, to get around the suffering, to achieve societies' definition of success. To be completely honest, my business and family success has been great. I've worked hard to get to where I am today and I'm really proud of the work ethic I have. But I'm still searching for ways to improve myself. There is always the next course, the next training, the next move, the next big thing to strive for. This is not bad. Expansion, growth, and learning are natural parts of human evolution. Growth is the most important thing there is.

Here is the key question you honestly have to ask yourself. Is your growth mindset coming from a sense that something is missing, or of not being good enough?

"One of the innermost beliefs most people have is, 'I'm not good enough. We frequently can add to that, I don't do enough, or I don't deserve.'"

—Louise L. Hay

If this is a new question for you, great! Asking yourself about what motivates your growth mindset is a starting point that can provide you with insights into why you do the things you do—into why you are motivated or not, and what drives you to accomplish the things you do. It's the first step in determining what's most important to you and why. For example, maybe you have the thought, "When I complete that course, I'll be taken seriously in my professional career,", or "once I finish that training, I'll be able to start my own business." Once I have "x," I'll finally be good enough to do "y."

Example:

As a _____, I'm expected to achieve_____ by _____ years of age or within a certain timeline.

In my own career, age was always a factor. I started my business when I was only twenty-three, so I thought people wouldn't take me seriously unless I dressed a certain way, spoke a certain way, or ran my business a certain way. I felt I was always trying to prove my worth by achieving more. My thoughts were, "When I am older, I'll be taken seriously, and my clients and business associates will respect me more." Behind that thought was, "I'm not good enough as I am now, but one day I will be."

There are so many external pressures and comparisons that can leave you feeling not good enough. This mindset of over-achieving to fill yourself up will eventually lead to the exact opposite—an empty tank and burnout or perhaps a health crisis that stops you in your tracks.

Luckily, there's a solution. Consider how your energy could shift if you approached growth and achievement from a space of "I am enough exactly as I am." Whether I take that course or not, whether I exercise today or not, whether I land that contract or not, whether someone acknowledges me or not, whether I'm twenty, forty, or sixty years old, I am perfectly enough exactly as I am.

This mindset can enhance not only the learning process, but also your ability to discover fulfillment in the here and now. Your growth will become part of a natural evolution rather than another part of you that needs fixing. This will eliminate the illusion of failure. If you could absolutely not fail, how would that influence your choice and change the way you show up for yourself and others? In hindsight, I can see that the limiting belief I held, that age was a determinant of success, was completely untrue. At the age of twenty-three, I was able to build my business to a level of success that allows me a comfortable lifestyle today. Age is only one limiting belief, and there are many others. What limiting belief are you managing by constantly working to achieve?

REFLECTION

1. What's possible if you approach any new task from, "I am enough with or without this _____"?

2. What courses or classes could you take for pure pleasure and enjoyment?

3. What are you passionate about not because it will advance your career or gain you more recognition but because it excites you?

DISGUISE #4: PROCRASTINATION

I've been procrastinating writing this section about procrastination. Why? Because what if I get it wrong? What if I don't have much to say about procrastination? Perhaps I should do more research, browse the web, and come back later? The truth is that the things we keep shelving for later are really the areas of our life that need the most attention and that we don't want to examine, commit to, follow through with, or finish up. Fear of failure, fear of being judged, fear of change, and fear of disappointment are a few examples of what may be true for you when you fall into the procrastination trap.

The word vulnerability continues to come to mind when I think about procrastination. I will often put things off that may require me to feel exposed or vulnerable. For example, I write a blog for my business once a month. I have thirty days to write a two-to-three paragraph blog, yet I continually wait until the last couple of days to write it. I feel like it has to be perfect, and that my energy has to feel just right before I sit down to write. I have to have a coffee, no interruptions, and feel inspired.

The environment will never be perfect for me to begin writing, until there's a hard deadline, like tomorrow, staring me in the face. This has been a pattern throughout my life. I tell myself that I do my best work under the pressure of deadlines. When I was in university, I was the one racing to finish the project the night before, often working after midnight, or studying the night before until moments before the exam. I wouldn't recommend this. It caused me so much stress—panicking late one night as my printer ran out of ink while printing off my final project. (Yes, that was before it was possible to submit assignments electronically.)

It's human nature to put off doing the things that we're unsure of. Perhaps you think you're not really good at a task or haven't perfected it, or maybe it's a task that you simply just don't like to do—like cleaning the fridge. You may be thinking, "But Laura, I really don't like to clean the house, organize the garage, clean out the basement," or whatever you fill in the blank with. That really is the end of the story. I still encourage you to dig a little deeper and ask yourself why you have been putting it off. Keep asking yourself *why* until you discover the root of your procrastination.

For me, procrastination is often rooted in the fear of not doing something perfectly. If I cannot fully complete the project with a perfectly polished outcome, in a certain amount of time, then I just won't even start. This is not just with writing a blog. It flows out into other aspects of my life like mopping the floors. I hate mopping floors, so it's the last thing I'll do because it takes time, and if I can't clean the entire house perfectly, then why do it at all? Perfection is a showstopper, a block. It stems from a fear of not doing something right and judging yourself for the imperfection.

Many other factors also contribute to procrastination:

- not knowing how to do something
- not having enough time to fully complete the task
- fear of being judged or criticized by others when the task is completed
- fear of being wrong
- boredom—if I complete this task, I won't know what to do next

Overcoming Procrastination: Create Habits

It's not easy to put yourself out there. It takes courage to take action when you don't know what the outcome will be. The action of creating habits will help if you struggle with procrastination. Habits are formed when you implement daily routines to help you accomplish the things that are most important to you. You may find that some things you thought were so important and always on your mind to accomplish, actually weren't that important. I like to divide my goals up into timelines.

Daily goals

What needs to be done every day? For me, it's exercise, meditation, yoga, writing, and drinking eight glasses of water. These activities are so important for my physical and mental well-being that they have become non-negotiables. I do them every day and usually at the same time. Your non-negotiables may be different, depending on your goals and interests. Regardless of what they are, plan to do them daily.

Short and long-term goals

I had a plan to clear all the old stuff from my basement. But every time I went down there, the amount of work overwhelmed me. That was two years ago. I talked about it with colleagues and my husband. It was on my mind constantly, yet I never took action. I started to feel bad about it because I was failing at this one task that I deemed important. Why was I procrastinating? Because the task felt too big to handle by myself. I worried that I couldn't do it, that I would fail. I was worried that I would do it wrong and throw out things of sentimental value that I would later regret. Perhaps this task would need a more fixed timeline.

Is there a task you'd like to accomplish that will take quite some time, that you can't finish in a weekend? (I like to think most tasks can be completed over a weekend—my poor husband!) Here's a strategy for turning procrastination into action:

1. Set up a realistic completion date for the project.
2. Set daily or weekly action steps you need to take to finish the task by the completion date.

3. Enlist support. Who do you need to assist you? If you have young kids, arrange a babysitter once a week to give yourself time. Ask your significant other to take something off your to-do list. Make whatever arrangements you need to complete what is important to you.

4. Adjust your plans if you need to. The best laid plans need room for flexibility. Notice whether you've created an unrealistic timeline. You may start off feeling excited and then end up feeling overwhelmed with the expectations you set. Be kind and compassionate with yourself and keep moving forward.

Procrastination is simply a habit you have created, but it is a habit that keeps you in stagnation. To break this habit, you'll need to start some new productive habits. Watch out for things or people that will distract you and fear that could be holding you back. Over time, the cognitive load of having to "think" about what you need to do next will lessen as the new habit becomes cemented. The new habit will become a part of you and your daily routine. What will follow are results. If you're wondering, I finally got that basement cleared out; —it only took two years. I'm now ready for the next step—creating a new more enjoyable space for exercising and relaxing. I feel much lighter and ready to move onto the next project!

REFLECTION

1. What will happen if you don't take action on the things that are important to you?

2. What outcomes are possible if you just start the project? Just begin by taking one step without worrying about the next step.

3. What is one task, project, or bucket list dream that you have spent so much time thinking about but have yet to take action? What is one action you could take TODAY to begin?

DISGUISE # 5: THE ILLUSION OF CONTROL

When I interview candidates for a job, I ask them, "How much of your life do you feel you control?" The answers I have gotten vary, from little control to total control. It's a bit of a trick question because there's no right or wrong answer. What I'm most curious about is if they believe they have an internal or external locus of control. A person with an internal locus of control believes their actions directly affect the results and outcomes. They believe the decisions they make, the work they do, and the effort they put forth will create the result they want. Someone with an external locus of control believes the outcomes of their lives are determined by external factors. They believe there's very little they can do to create the outcomes they desire.

Typically, people fall somewhere on the continuum between internal and external. It's an important area to examine as you start to become more intentional in creating a life you desire. Discovering where you land on the continuum can provide great insight as we move forward. With this awareness, you can find harmony between taking aligned right actions while learning to detach from the outcome and lean into faith that your path will unfold in its perfection.

There are many things that occur in the external environment that you have no control over. A natural disaster, a war on the other side of the world, interest rates, the price of gas. If you take time to stop and observe the space around you, you will notice constant change. Our external environment and even our own bodies are in constant motion. Everything is moving energy. Many things may be out of your control but how you choose to react and shift with the changing environment is within your power.

Our fears can be triggered by physical events like skydiving, swimming, public speaking, or flying on an airplane. Other times an emotional threat that challenges our sense of self and our beliefs can also bring fear to the surface. Being out of control is a common fear, so we do our best to put practices in place that give us a feeling of safety and comfort. This could look like trying to control another person or putting more constraints and rules in place that we think will favour a particular outcome.

Although certain actions may increase our odds of success, there is no guarantee. (Read more on this in Chapter 7.) The illusion that we are in control can temporarily make us feel good, but it doesn't last. As soon as another threat or trigger occurs, the cycle begins again until the attempt to control begins to block you from trusting the universe and the natural flow of life. When this happens, challenges and struggles are amplified. You end up always bumping up against apparent obstacles. Instead of seeing the opportunity to shift with the change, you fight and fight.

Blocked flow =
stress, dis-ease in the body, conflict in the mind, challenge
in relationships, anger, complaining, low energy, a sense
of unrest

Here is a typical path of reactivity:

1. An external event occurs—trigger.

2. This triggering event brings up a thought or belief that elicits a fear response.

3. The protective part of you reacts unconsciously in an attempt to fix *or* defend what feels scary and out of your control.

This reaction often propels you into action—over-planning to quell your fears and/or enlisting others who agree with you to justify your actions.

This is the typical loop that can play many times a day without your awareness. You become the "fixer" of situations that threaten your comfort in some way. The problem is that any fixes that come from a place of fear and anxiety will only be temporary.

Inspirational speaker and spiritual teacher Wayne Dyer promoted this principle: "You cannot solve a problem with the same mind that created it." As soon as the next threat comes along, the process starts all over again.

Have you ever wondered why similar situations seem to repeat themselves in your life—even if you move, change jobs, leave an unhealthy relationship? It's because you've found a temporary solution, —like putting a bandage on a bleeding wound. Unless the wound is healed, it will continue to bleed no matter where you go. We are often too busy with the doing and fixing that we don't take the time to stop and listen to what is really buried beneath the surface.

One of my fears is getting sick when I travel because I feel out of control in a different environment (triggering event, plus old belief) I try to control this fear by being prepared (attempt to fix the problem). I believe that if I'm prepared enough, I won't get sick, so I start taking all kinds of immune boosters the week before I go on a trip. Then I pack every single remedy in our medicine cabinet—from Advil, Pepto Bismol, Band-Aids, and oregano oil, to hand sanitizer for the airplane--overplanning to quell the fear.

When I travel with my kids, it's even worse. I try so hard to control not being sick, that I often get sick or someone in my family does. I take so much time and energy focusing on illness and trying to control the next week to ten days that I believe I manifest sickness. Focusing on the worst possible outcome to get out ahead of it usually lands you right in the outcome you were trying to avoid.

Now when I notice this fear of being out of control arising, I use the steps from Chapter 1 and challenge the belief.

1. Triggering thought: I'm travelling to a different country on an airplane with hundreds of other people. I'm definitely going to get sick and won't have access to medical help. I ask myself, "IS THIS TRUE?" The answer is no; this is not the absolute truth.

2. Replace this thought/belief with, "I take good care of myself physically, spiritually, and mentally. My immune system is strong, and I have the support I need in every moment.

3. Mantras: "I am healthy." "I am fully supported by the universe and have everything I need in the moment." "All is well."

4. I repeat the mantra as often as needed, especially when I observe the triggering thought occurring in my day-to-day life.

Instead of worrying about an outcome, which is really a stream of anxious thoughts, you can trust that you'll have everything you need in that moment to get through whatever comes up. You can apply these steps to any area of your life where fear is causing you to grip in an effort to control the outcome. Finding a balance between being prepared and trusting the universe to support you is the key to moving forward with ease.

It's easy to write this and to logically understand how letting go of the illusion of control is good for us, but how can we actually do that on a regular basis?

Surrender

> *"You are afraid of surrender because you don't want to lose control, but you never had control; all you had was anxiety."*
>
> —Elizabeth Gilbert

I don't love the word surrender, because for me it triggers a feeling of defeat, of giving up control under duress. In the Merriam-Webster dictionary, it means "to give (something) over to the control or possession of another usually under duress." The word has a negative connotation because that's what we've been taught. *But now consider how giving up the need to control outcomes is in fact giving up your own anxiety.* Surrender then begins to take on a new feeling of peace and ease.

When you first start to practise surrender it may feel like you're giving up, like you're not doing everything in your power to get the result you want. But that doesn't mean you don't take action. On the contrary, you take action based on the facts—the information you have available in the moment and from a place of pure trust. The information will change, sometimes minute to minute, hour to hour, week to week. You will change. Your needs, desires, and wants will shift. Nothing is stagnant in our moving universe, not even you. I can't tell you the number of ideas, and goals that I've changed or completely thrown out. I've either learned more and decided to change my course of action or, after some time, I realized the idea was no longer a fit for what was most important to me at that time.

Learning to be malleable when the world is constantly shifting will have an immediate impact on your physical and mental well-being and strengthen your resilience (more in Chapter 7). The act of surrender releases you from trying to solve all the problems of the world. When this state prevails within you, solutions will come to you. You will be in a better state to flow with whatever comes your way.

Practising Presence

There are many ways to practise presence. Here are a few that I love.

1. **Immerse yourself in nature.** Go for a walk or a hike in the woods, ski, swim, lie in the grass, sit in the sun, and observe nature—the trees, the wind, the grass, the birds, the squirrels, the sky. Watch the sunrise or sunset. Observing nature naturally brings you into alignment with the present moment. Nature does not lie. It is the purest representation of truth. You can trust it, and when you fully trust, you can surrender.

2. **Practise yoga.** Yoga requires you to concentrate on your physical body in time and space. Yes, your mind will drift, but the sensations you feel in your body will guide you back to the present moment. Practising yoga has taught me that the more I hold on and try to control the physical poses, the harder it is. It's only when I exhale and surrender that my body begins to soften and move more freely. Practising the act of surrender on the yoga mat will help you to discover how this can feel off your mat.

3. **Practise focused awareness.** Make a conscious decision to be present in the actions you are making physically when doing a task. I like to choose simple tasks that have become habits like doing the dishes, folding laundry, cutting the grass, vacuuming, and driving. Notice the texture of what you are touching, the temperature of the room, the beating of your heart, your breath moving in and out. By focusing on the physical, you can move your awareness into the present and away from the racing thoughts that can be a source of worry and concern.

REFLECTION

1. Think of an area of your life that you like to control. If you loosened the reins of control, how would you feel? What fears do you have of letting go in this area?

2. Is there a payoff for maintaining control and managing your fear? For example, when I over-pack medications on my vacations, I feel like I'm taking charge of my health and I'm prepared. The payoff is that I feel safe because I've created a sense of security.

3. What's possible if you acknowledge the fear, choose courage, and do it anyway? What's the best outcome you can imagine?

FEAR IS NOT BAD

Fear is a signal that some part of your life or situation needs attention.

Fear triggers can be used as a guide for growth. When fear is present, there is an opportunity to look deeper at the situation. Hiding, controlling, manipulating, and masking your discomforts keeps the fear alive. When you are aware of your fears and can meet them with compassion and courage, the hold they have on you will begin to soften. For example, for many people, just thinking about public speaking triggers fear, yet thousands of people do it every day—they practise being with their fear and doing it anyway. I challenge you to find one public speaker who doesn't get just a bit nervous before they take the stage.

When I teach yoga—I've been doing it for about six years—I get really flushed and hot, not because I don't feel confident as a teacher, but because I fear the class won't be good enough. I'm afraid that someone won't like the class, that I'll be judged, so my nervous system responds with a physical reaction.

There's a concept I speak about when I teach yoga:

When you experience a yoga pose that's uncomfortable and challenging, you can choose to stay in the pose, trusting that you will get through it and be even stronger. The moment you want to quit, come out of the pose, run the other way, is the moment of a new breakthrough, if you stay.

I strive to embody this concept when I teach a class, run my business, develop a workshop, or try new things. Stay in the pose until you can relax into it, breathe, and surrender to what is. Soften your face and shoulders, and just breathe with ease. Facing uncomfortable situations involves staying with and getting through the discomfort to the other side where there is ease. It's the same as facing fear. Fear presents itself, and you stay and breathe and soften and keep going with gentle ease. You let the fear happen, and by sitting with it, you find out what is on the other side. The more you practise, the less hold the fear will have on you.

Growth = Noticing the fear and doing it anyway

The goal is to shorten the time between the fear trigger and your awareness of it. This takes practice and can sometimes take multiple attempts to get your attention. But believe me, the universe will send you situations, people, or circumstances that will trigger your fear again. Don't run from them. These situations may make you uncomfortable and can be challenging. Life is not planned and organized. It is chaotic, changing, exciting, inspiring, and full of unknown possibilities and opportunities. I would love to have a life with nothing out of place, perfect in every way. Many of us strive for this, but total order and predictability are not practical. There is no amount of planning, organizing, or perfecting that can collision-proof your life.

We've been fooled into believing that if we do the "right" things, the challenging times can be avoided. But growth happens during challenging times. It's easy to be happy, loving, joyful and supportive when things are going well. But how do you react when things are not going well? When you lose a job or a loved one or your freedom, how do you react? Your reaction is the only thing you can control.

Can you be aware enough to stay in the moment? Can you be aware enough to see the lesson—shorten the length of time between reaction and awareness? This awareness will help bring you out of the automatic fear response and enable you to choose a more supportive response.

If you are in physical danger or harm, do your best to remove yourself from the situation- Call for help and find support. The intention of the above section is to highlight the mental fears we conjure up in our mind when there is no threat of imminent physical danger.

"95% of our thoughts arise from programs in the sub-conscious mind"

— Bruce Lipton

CHAPTER 3

CREATING A NEW STORY

BELIEFS

Bruce Lipton, a stem cell biologist, and bestselling author of *Biology of Belief,* has spent his life researching the effects of thoughts and beliefs on genetic expression and quality of life. He surmises that we operate from our conscious minds, creative wishes, and desires only five per cent of the day. The other ninety-five per cent of our thoughts, beliefs and actions arise from programs in our subconscious mind.

The subconscious mind is programmed between birth and age seven. This is when the brain is primarily in theta frequency, a state between wakefulness and sleep that relates to the subconscious mind. According to NeuroHealth Associates, theta brainwaves are strong during times of internal focus, meditation, prayer, and spiritual awareness. This state is not typical in awake adults but is normal while we sleep and in children up to age seven.

This theta state is like being in a state of hypnosis and allows children to absorb a tremendous amount of information from their environment. The environment consists of who we spend most of our time with, namely, parents or caretakers, teachers, siblings, friends, social groups and teams, and the culture we grow up in.

The information that is absorbed becomes the baseline for a set of beliefs that get stored in the subconscious mind, similar to the operating system of a computer. This allows us to perform functions we need to without having to consciously think about them.

Here's the problem: since these beliefs are subconscious, the conscious wishes and desires you have are no match for the ninety-five per cent of the time that your brain is operating from a set of beliefs that were established many years ago. You may want to make a change, but established blocks continue to manifest, and you remain in the pattern. Subconscious beliefs can also be problematic in relationships because each person brings their own unconscious beliefs to the table.

A simple example illustrates how subconscious beliefs work. When you date someone for a long time, you think you have a pretty good idea of their beliefs and behaviours. You decide to move in together, but sharing a living space is very different and can be eye opening. By joining two households, you're meshing a lifetime of learned beliefs. Gender-based beliefs are especially influenced by our parents and culture. These beliefs become imprinted by observing the dynamics within our families of origin; for example, who does the laundry, cooking, cleaning, grass cutting, repairs, shopping. If your beliefs are similar, the transition will be smooth. If not, it can be a rocky road.

Not all partners, friends, co-workers, or other people we have relationships with share the same beliefs. For example, we all have beliefs about how our kids should behave, how our partner should treat us, how our co-workers should work within the team—essentially how the world should be according to our beliefs. Becoming aware of the core beliefs that influence your life and your decisions is very liberating.

Awareness is the first step toward making real, lasting change. If you're unaware, how can you seek to make improvements? You can start by simply observing your life—your job, family, social life, passions, income, home, daily routines—your entire life as it is right now. Notice what areas of your life are not working as you would like them to. What areas are you struggling in?

The beliefs that were programmed into you by age seven play out in your daily life. Some beliefs are supportive and help you to create a life of joy and fulfillment. Other beliefs may cast a negative shadow and deter you from manifesting your desires. We call these limiting beliefs. You can start to make changes in your life when you become witness to how your beliefs are a series of learned concepts about how the world should be.

Some beliefs we hold may appear minor. For example, one belief I have is that my husband should take out the trash on garbage day, but that doesn't mean he should. It is what I witnessed as a child: Dad took out the garbage every week, and when my brother got older, it became his job. It is a gender-based belief that I learned. The roles of men and women vary greatly across families and cultures.

Other beliefs we hold will carry more weight and will therefore carry more influence on the direction of your life. For example, a self-limiting belief for me that often creeps into my reality is that I'm not ready or not experienced enough. This belief holds me back from taking chances and doing something new.

It is not an absolute truth that your belief is right, and another is wrong, although it really feels absolute in the moment. It is when we are in our "rightness" that we get into arguments and disputes in our relationships with others and on an even greater scale, with other nations and cultures.

There are, of course, some absolute truths such as the existence of gravity—whether you believe in gravity or not, this invisible force is real. Aside from proven fact, however, your belief system is rooted in your own experiences and upbringing. Through them, you draw conclusions about how the world is or, more directly, how the world is perceived by you.

True freedom comes from making choices for yourself from a place of greater awareness and clarity. Your beliefs have become a guide for you in navigating all the decisions you have made so far in your life. As your awareness grows, you will realize that some of your programmed beliefs really don't work for you anymore. The great news is that you can change them if you want to. And you can keep the beliefs that do work. The important takeaway is to be malleable, open, and curious about what you believe and why.

Our truest of truths is limited only by what we believe right now, today, to be true. This is captured in a quote that I love: *"You don't know what you don't know."*

For example, science is ever evolving. Humans used to believe the world was flat. We used to believe that solid things were made of solid materials. Now we know that everything in this world is made up of particles that are moving at different rates. And beyond moving particles, quantum physics has taught us that atoms viewed at their subatomic size become energy waves of pure frequency. Everything in our physical world is made up of waves and frequency—pure energy.

What we believed about our world 100 years ago is very different from what we believe now. And decades from now, what we believe will be drastically different. Did people in 1901 ever think it would be possible to communicate over an invisible frequency we call Wi-Fi? The idea of a World Wide Web would have been crazy. Scientific truth will continue to change as measuring tools evolve, and as new hypotheses and experiments form. Can you bring this fervour of curiosity to your own beliefs and know they can and will shift and change, either naturally or with intent?

REFLECTION

1. Choose one belief you have about yourself that holds you back from making a change.

2. Is this belief absolutely true? How do you know?

3. If this belief is not absolutely true, how would this change your perspective and choices?

4. Rewrite an old belief from the new perspective of possibility.

ATTRACTOR PATTERNS

I grew up with everything you could ever ask for—a loving home, a great neighbourhood, lots of friends, and parents who enjoyed family trips and hosting fun family parties. My parents were also entrepreneurs and change makers in a way that was unique from other parents I knew. When I was about ten years old, my mom started travelling to Africa with a mission to do charity work in Tanzania, Africa, often leaving for a month or two at a time. My dad was a teacher with a passion for developing new businesses. He also loved sports, so he started a basketball league in our area that is still going strong forty-five years later.

Clearly, I had very busy, entrepreneurial parents who taught me the values of hard work, commitment, and giving back to the community. For the most part, as a child, I was content to be on my own. I had three siblings, but two were a bit older and didn't really want to hang out with their little sister, so my younger childhood memories consist mostly of me and my brother, who was a year younger.

At ten years old, I didn't fully understand the depth of my parents' work. I was often left on my own and learned to be quite independent. My story or attractor pattern became, "I am alone. People I love leave me to do other important things, and there-fore I am not important enough." Although this was not true, my young mind interpreted it as true, and it became a subconscious belief pattern that I was unaware of at the time.

The first time I remember this story showing up in my life was in Grade 5 when one of my best friends moved away. I had been a shy, quiet child, so it wasn't always easy making new friends. Yet, I desperately wanted to fit in, be cool, outgoing, and have lots of friends. One day, a new student arrived in our class, and I was determined to become friends with her. And I did—in fact, we became great friends! We had sleepovers, played on the same basketball team, hung out at recess, and ate lunch together. Then after two years she and her family moved three hours away.

For a twelve-year-old, this is very far away. I was really upset. We promised to write and call, and we did for about a year. My parents even drove me to my friend's new house so we could spend the weekend skiing together. But then her dad changed jobs again and the family moved to Michigan, a ten-hour drive away. We continued to write and talk, but slowly it became less and less. By high school we had drifted apart completely.

I didn't know it at the time, but I took the situation very personally. I missed my friend dearly and I felt left behind, unimportant, and alone. These feelings of aloneness continued to manifest in other situations in my life where people I loved, people I depended on and trusted, left me. This program ran in my subconscious mind at a level that required no attention from me, continuing to attract similar situations.

I wasn't aware of this pattern until my mid-thirties when I began to do the self-reflective work in my yoga teacher training. I slowly saw how this program continued to play out in my life. This program played unconsciously on repeat until it moved from my subconscious into my conscious awareness.

An attractor pattern works like this:

1. You hold a subconscious belief that you are unaware of.

2. This belief acts like a magnet that pulls situations to you that reinforce the belief: even if there's another viewpoint, you will see what you believe about the situation.

3. Your conscious mind may want something different so there is a dissonance between what is happening and what you wanted to have happen.

4. The present situation dissolves: you may even forget about it. Move on.

5. The same pattern emerges from this belief and begins to repeat itself in another experience.

This cycle repeats itself and becomes a recurring pattern in your life. You may feel frustrated and hopeless that the same thing happens repeatedly with different people, a different job, or different place.

The big question then becomes, how do you stop attracting things to you that you don't want? The answer is simple, but the practice will require a concentrated, consistent effort from you.

Nothing changes unless you change. You will continue to attract the same type of relationships, jobs, crises, or problems until you begin to recognize you are the common denominator in all the situations. This is not to create shame. This is how the brain, and the law of attraction works. Until you are aware that you are the epicentre of your experiences and perceptions, there is absolutely no way you can change it. You have the capacity to change your circumstances by shifting your perceptions. If you want to create a new job, a better relationship with yourself, your spouse, or your family, you can. If you accept responsibility for the role you play in creating your life, you can then get excited knowing that you get to choose how the next chapter will unfold.

Bruce Lipton describes three ways to change subconscious beliefs:

1. **New habits**: Repetition of a new supportive narrative will help to re-form beliefs (mantras/affirmations). This may take time and require you to be hyperaware of your patterns and beliefs.

2. **Hypnosis:** During hypnosis, your brain dips into the theta state. By bringing the brain into this state, you can re-program new thoughts and beliefs into the subconscious mind. This is a faster, more direct way to shift belief patterns.

3. **Energy psychology:** A much faster results-oriented process for reprogramming the brain as it taps into the electrical energy systems of the body—the heart, nervous system, energy meridians and the biofield. Subconscious programming can be shifted immediately as a new program is put in its place.

I began by practising a new narrative and then by engaging in hypnotherapy. Slowly, as I became the observer of a repetitive pattern, I started to catch myself in the middle of the thought or belief that was fueling it. I would come back to the present moment and ask myself, "Is it true? Am I unimportant and alone? Am I taking this personally? Maybe it has nothing to do with me. This would immediately create a shift in the belief pattern, and it would begin to dissolve in that moment of awareness. I was able to become a witness to my reactions and to the pattern I was attracting.

I eventually learned that the only thing that was telling me I was not important was the program from my subconscious mind. Until I could reprogram my mind that I was important and supported, the pattern would continue. It wasn't me who was unimportant; rather, it was my interpretation, or perception, of the situation from the lens of an old belief. I was taking things very personally. When I let this old belief go, a great burden was lifted. I realized that every single person on this planet is important, including me. And every single person is on their own journey, having the experience they came here to have. I let go of taking things personally. I changed the narrative and, eventually, the belief.

The Payoff of Attractor Patterns

Another reason for repeating patterns showing up in your life is the payoff. I always choose to be busy so I can feel productive and not lazy. I am always moving from one task to the next and find it difficult to sit down and relax. In my subconscious mind, I'm only good enough when I'm being productive. The payoff is that I feel good about myself when I get things done. It masks the deeper belief that I'm not enough unless I'm doing something productive. It's like taking ibuprofen for a headache. It stops the pain temporarily, but the source of the pain is still there.

And so, believing that my productivity is connected to my self-worth harms my physical and mental health. I get worn out, tired, stressed, and overwhelmed, and my creative output drops when I am too busy. Yet I still focus on being productive because there is a payoff of temporarily feeling good. To be clear, there is nothing wrong with feeling good for completing tasks and contributing to your family, workplace, or community. The trouble arises when this pattern becomes a measure of your worthiness: without the accomplishment you're not good enough. But your worthiness is your birthright—you are worthy because you are here now. Even if you contribute less one day—you don't make an amazing meal for your family, don't do the laundry, don't cut the grass—you are still worthy.

As you begin this work of becoming aware of your beliefs, keep asking yourself, why you do what you do. Begin by looking at an area of your life where you feel overwhelmed, exhausted or are unhappy with the results, and keep asking yourself why you are so overextended. Why do you choose to _____? The answers will reveal themselves when you start to ask and get quiet enough to listen.

Thoughts and beliefs, like emotions, are pure energy. You can choose to follow them, or you can let them pass by. You can choose to believe them or not. True freedom is having the choice to believe or not believe.

REFLECTION

1. Is there somewhere in your life where you see a pattern on repeat?

2. What belief is fueling that pattern?

3. If you could interrupt that pattern and observe the thought, what lie is it telling you over and over again?

4. What is the payoff for believing in this lie? In other words, what do you get out of allowing this thought to direct your life?

STORIES AND THE EGO

Wherever you go, there you are.

When you were born, you arrived without an ego, or without a concept of I, me, and mine. When we're babies, the self-concept is not yet developed. There's no separation between where we came from and our "selves." Naturally, we grow in a world that has been divided into polar opposites—good and evil, loud and quiet, happy and sad, young and old, smart and not so smart. So, it's completely normal that we begin to identify with the world in separate parts. We eventually find our place in this world as defined by finite walls influenced by gender, race, social status, wealth, parents divorced or still married or no parents, being adopted, having siblings, or not having siblings, being religious or not religious. These walls are the beginning of our story.

We all have a story and within this story is the main character, which you call *you* or *me*. Your sense of self is known as your ego. There is nothing wrong with the ego self. We all have one. In fact, the ego plays an important role in creating the drive to move toward your desires, dreams and goals. Ego is an important part of being human. Yet over time, and as a natural result of conditioning and daily living, we come to completely self-identify with the ego. It becomes *you* so strongly that you forget your true Self.

Imagine you are watching a really good movie. The movie hooks your attention so much that you feel the emotions of the characters as if you were in the movie. You forget the crunch of popcorn around you, you forget you're sitting in a dark theatre with a hundred other people and for a brief time, you forget about your outside life. At the end of the movie, the lights come on, the credits roll, and you come back to your life and your body. You know you are not the movie or part of the movie. You are the observer of the movie.

This is exactly what happens with your ego self. Your life is the movie, and you are the star. With all its ups and downs and twists and turns, your movie is pretty exciting. You are so identified with it that you believe you are the movie. You become so lost in it that you forget about the part of you that is watching the movie—the observer, the true Self.

You've been building your story since your ego began to emerge. Your story is helpful because it compartmentalizes concepts and we as humans function better in a defined environment. When we interact with our physical environment in a divisive way, it allows us to process and interact in the physical world. We begin to fit in. Our story then begins to keep us safe, comfortable, and part of a predictable routine.

On the flip side, the story you've created is also confining and restricts you to one way of being in the world. You get stuck in a pattern. This pattern begins to define who you are and becomes a great reason for justifying your behaviour, like "I do this because this is how I was raised." Your story becomes so much a part of you that it blocks you from seeing a new path and new opportunities for growth and change.

For example, a person who likes to be spontaneous, take risks, and try new things may describe themselves as adventurous and their friends and family may expect them to always be this way. If that person then chooses a different path, to be more conservative and cautious, for example, their new way of being is considered unusual.

If you continue to let your story define you, you will make choices that support that part of your story. But if that story is holding you back from accomplishing what you truly desire, it's time to change it. Begin by examining where you are limiting yourself. Once you can step back and become the observer, you then have the choice to stay in the story or create a new one. Your true power shines when you know you have a choice. By repeating a new supportive pattern or habit, you can empower yourself and move into more conscious, balanced action, creating a life you truly desire.

Transcending The Ego

In my current story, I'm a woman, a mother, a business owner, a wife, a daughter, a sister, a friend, and a yoga instructor. I define myself as quiet, calm, and a bit of an introvert. I don't like speaking in front of groups, I'm not that adventurous, and I don't like to take uncalculated risks. There are many more ways I define myself, but this is the basic structure of my ego. This has been my story for a long time. It has allowed me to build a comfortable life. I live in a great home, I am financially secure, I have a beautiful loving family, and I have a successful business. All of this is wonderful by external standards, yet I still craved more. I'd been living by the standard of what success and happiness should look like, so why wasn't it enough? Something was lacking and I knew there was more to life than these external markers of "success."

When you are no longer satisfied within your ego-defined self,
it is the true Self that is craving expansion.

The ego is constantly striving for more. It seeks accolades, rewards, and a pat on the back when you win. The ego is never satisfied with being where it is. When outside success no longer satisfies you, it's time to look deeper to explore the limits you've placed on yourself, that which are containing your expansion and evolution.

I had let my ego take over and define my story. I had forgotten about the observer, my true Self, my Soul, where I had come from, and where I will return to one day. I had forgotten what truths mattered to me—love, peace, harmony, compassion, and joy. I had forgotten that no matter what my story was or where it was taking me, if these five truths were missing, then my true Self was missing. My ego had taken the reins.

You can change your story and expand beyond your perceived limitations, but if the ego is the only part of you steering the ship, you will arrive at your new destination disappointed and searching once again for more. Become aware of your story, notice how it confines you, make changes if necessary, but remember to take your true Self along for the ride. The observer is the true Self that wants nothing more than to expand in love and peace.

Foggy Glasses

Imagine viewing the world since you were born through a pair of foggy glasses. You would think this is how the world looks and will always look. One day, a wise person approaches you and notices your glasses are very foggy. They offer you a new pair, a new perspective. You try them on hesitantly because these foggy glasses are all you've ever known. They have been a part of who you are, and you don't want to give them up. They fit well, they're comfortable, stylish, and they've served you well up until now.

But there are some things you haven't been able to do with your foggy glasses, so you decide to try on the new glasses. When you do, your entire view changes. The grass looks greener, the sky more blue, the flowers pop with colour. You're astonished that there was so much you were missing with your foggy, well-intentioned, comfortable glasses.

These foggy glasses are your story. You view the world through the confines of the story that society, parents, teachers, and the media have told you about who you are and who you are supposed to be. I know this, because I continue to witness my never-ending inner dialogue that has opinions on who I should be, how I should feel, and how I should act in order to keep my story alive.

Inside the story, there is a feeling of known safety because on some level it works for you and has brought you this far in your life. It takes a tremendous amount of courage to challenge your story and break free of its limitations. No one way of being is ever finite. Each day, each hour, each moment is different. There is fluidity to our moods, thoughts, emotions, and beliefs.

Changing the story can be challenging when you are in familiar situations and around the same people, especially people who have known you for a long time. Your story gets reinforced by how people who know you well expect you to act. It's a very common trap to get caught in but the more you practise and question the status quo of the life you have created, the more you can expand your views and find greater fulfillment.

There's a part of me that will always crave expansion and growth—to be better than I was yesterday, and to learn more about myself and others and the exciting dance we call life. Having a growth mindset will lead you to experience greater fulfillment in your day-to-day life. It will encourage you to challenge the status quo. When you find it's more difficult to stay in the story you have created, it will be invaluable to continue to ask yourself what you truly want and why. This will help you gain clarity on what is most important (see Chapter 5). It's a huge relief when you begin to remove the blocks that have held you back. The right people show up at the right time. New opportunities begin to arise. You start to see things that you've never seen before. Each new awakening leads softly to the next.

You may experience struggles along the way and your confidence will be challenged as it often is when starting something new. Remember, you are really good at being in your story. You've practised it every day for years. Trying out new ways of being can feel messy, disorganized, and awkward—and not like you are being yourself at all. When you start to change, the people that know you best may not like it. You are a character in their story too, so when you begin to act in new, unpredictable ways, their comfortable story also begins to change, and you may have to renegotiate the terms of your relationship with them, kindly and patiently. Communicate your wants, needs and dreams to those closest to you. Share your goals and ask for support. Having a support team makes the process of transformation go all that more smoothly.

REFLECTION

1. Write out your story. Who are you, what do you do, what's your personality, what do you like and dislike?

2. What parts of your story stop you from taking action towards a goal?

3. How have you let others define you? For example, are you the one who always overreacts, who doesn't take chances, or who gives up on things?

4. Rewrite your story the way you want it to be.

TRUST THE JOURNEY: CHALLENGES ARE DETOURS IN THE RIGHT DIRECTION

Resistance doesn't change reality; it just makes it more difficult.

You are on a path, a journey that has twists and turns. Like a raging river, it's sometimes choppy and chaotic and may feel like there's no direction at all. And sometimes it's calm and peaceful and flowing almost effortlessly in a set direction. No matter where you are right now, in this moment you are steering the boat through the sea of your life. You are the captain—you have the power and freedom to decide how you want to navigate the situations that show up in your life.

This metaphor reminds me of sailing. Although I love the water and love to swim and explore new areas, particularly on water, sailing kind of scares me because I have only ever done it a couple of times. A few years back, my husband and I went to visit friends in British Columbia, Canada. They're seasoned sailors and wanted to take us out on their boat. I felt a little fearful. The ocean is unpredictable, and my inexperience meant I would not be able to control the situation- even though I have the tools to cope with this situation—fear is still a powerful emotion.

I like sailing when the wind is light, and the waves are small. It's gentle, peaceful, and relaxing, and you can take in the scenery without having to worry too much about hanging on for dear life when the waves and wind pick up. In these conditions, though, there's not much forward momentum. The calm, peaceful times when everything is going smoothly feel good: these are times when you can recharge and prepare for the wind.

Most sailors like strong winds blowing behind them that can catch the sail and move them quickly toward their destination. From what I observed, they get excited when the boat dips down and heels excessively toward the water. Although this forward momentum is quick, it isn't straight. You have to play the wind and tack up into it. This is when they make the fastest, forward progress. Challenges in your life are like strong winds that bump you off your path, but move you forward in a new direction. This is when the greatest growth occurs. Challenge builds resilience and strength and as you move forward you learn to make adjustments along the way.

During trying times, try to adjust your perspective and see how the challenges are happening *for* you, gently nudging you forward. No matter how you choose to see the wind, the change is still occurring. Resistance doesn't change reality, it just makes it more difficult. If you could choose a new perspective, you will fall into a more harmonious flow of your life. When you are in flow, you will know. Opportunities, people, and events show up for us almost without trying. Your life becomes synchronistic. In *Wisdom of the Oracle*, author and psychic medium Colette Baron-Reid explains: "Sometimes the synchronicity leads you directly into difficult situations in order to deliver an important lesson you need to learn" (p. 70).

In twenty years of running my business, I've had many synchronistic opportunities come my way—the right timing, the right support, the perfect opportunity. These opportunities felt like they were delivered on a silver platter. Not all came to fruition, but many did! Not all opportunities work out. The lesson here for me has always been "trust." Trust that the right opportunity will take hold and grow. If it doesn't, the effort is not lost nor wasted. It may not always be easy to accept the challenging times or the opportunities that slipped away, but how you decide to show up for the process is what matters. The real gift is the journey.

REFLECTION

1. Think back to a challenging time in your past. Looking back on it now, how did you grow and learn from it?

2. Is there a situation from your past that at the time was challenging but ended up leading to a better opportunity or outcome?

3. What tools can you lean on that will help to remind you of this during future challenging times?

"Knowing yourself is the beginning of all wisdom"

— Aristotle

CHAPTER 4

DISCOVERING YOUR TRUE SELF

When you start to peel back the layers of beliefs, thoughts, stories, attractor patterns and ego-centred thinking, you may wonder, if I am not my ego, who am I and—more importantly—how do I tap into my true Self?

CONSCIOUSNESS

Consciousness is about simply becoming aware—of our feelings, thoughts, beliefs, and perceptions. It's about waking up and taking notice. Your entire future is created from this present moment. In other words, what you plant today will continue to grow into the life you experience tomorrow. When you focus on what's not working, what will never work or how things are right now, you will create more of what you have. When you can take time to be present with your thoughts and beliefs, ultimately the emotions around your beliefs will be revealed. It's in the deeper layer of beliefs and emotions where all creation and manifestation begin. Even deeper, beyond that layer is where the true Self resides—the part of you that is always there, still, peaceful, silent, and calm, like the deepest part of the ocean. Some may call it your Soul. It is where pure potentiality and all possibility exist.

So how do you get to the deeper part of yourself—to this state of calm? On my journey of self-discovery, I often used my analytical mind to search for tangible steps to access this deeper part of myself, but what I learned was the harder I tried to "think," the more frustrated I would get. "Why am I not enlightened? Why are all these problems still happening to me? Why am I still feeling anxious, overwhelmed with not moving forward fast enough in my life? Why do I feel stuck?"

These thoughts would overwhelm me as I tried to meditate and find "Zen" and make my life happen. I began to realize that this push to tap into my true self was actually creating a barrier, not a path. Instead of the push forward, work hard mentality I grew up with, this inner work is softer. It's gradual and subtle, until one day you begin to notice that you feel more at ease, you have more patience, you worry less, you begin trusting more, new opportunities arise, the right people and resources show up. Your friends and family may even notice that something about you is different—and in a good way!

What I've discovered is that there really is no single formula for getting "there"; rather, there are tools you can use daily that help to cultivate a heightened state of consciousness.

Practise Self-Reflection

All of the self-reflection work you do is important. You cannot change what you do not see. These seemingly small steps lead to bigger moments of awakening that can come at any time. Each little moment is like a step up the ladder to experiencing freedom from that which holds you back. You are the one who holds the key to true freedom for yourself.

For a long time, I was looking outside myself for answers—to opinions from friends, family, experts, books, and podcasts. This type of support is helpful in gaining a new perspective and perhaps learning something new—but ultimately all the answers you seek are within you. With self-reflection, you can become aware of why you make certain decisions and begin to uncover the unconscious part of yourself that is really making the decisions. It's important to find some stillness each day, free from distraction, to reflect. This allows you to step out of unconsciously reacting to the events of your day. For me books, workshops, yoga, meditation, and speaking with like-minded friends have been helpful in guiding me to get in touch with my true Self. Becoming aware of your patterns is enough to cause awakening and change.

Notice Your Habits

The human brain is amazing. It takes in a ton of information in a day, and it chooses what it pays attention to and what it ignores. Research shows that when humans learn a new task, like driving a car or riding a bike, it takes a lot of brain power. Once we learn the mechanics and get really comfortable with the new skill, the subconscious takes over and it becomes second nature. We no longer have to pay attention to putting on the turn signal, or to the amount of pressure we put on the gas pedal. These actions become a habit. Forming habits are important because they lessen the cognitive load on our brain.

When your responses and behaviours become habits, you learn to predict responses and may think something like, "I just know how my spouse/partner/friend/boss will respond," or "I just know that when I do A the result will be B." When you've already figured out the answer before taking time to entertain a new possibility, you build a self-imposed fortress around you—meaning you've already predicted the outcome so there's no room for a new result. You may take your time with a decision and get advice from friends and family or make a quick in-the-moment decision, but ultimately you make the decision based on your past and the habits you have formed over a lifetime.

You know you're making habitual choices when the scenery is different (different people, places or events), but the experience feels similar. This is a massive clue that there is an underlying belief pattern running in your subconscious programming. Take notice of situations or obstacles that repeat over and over in your life and how you react or deal with them. This is where your habits will become crystal clear. Once you take notice, ask yourself, how could I respond or choose differently so perhaps a more supportive result occurs? Oftentimes, new and creative solutions will come to mind.

Keep a Journal

Journaling is powerful. A regular journaling routine allows you to get your steady stream of thoughts out onto paper. Whether to vent or simply work through a struggle, writing down your thoughts and feelings can be very therapeutic. Journaling can also offer a new perspective or solution to a problem, decision, or dilemma you are facing. I used to journal all the time until I "got too busy." This past year, the stress of the pandemic often left me feeling frustrated, agitated, and angry. So, I just began writing—about nothing and everything.

I used writing to vent, complain, and spew without fear that someone would read what I wrote and judge me for it. Now, journaling has become a place of pure, uncensored solace. It helps me to feel liberated from the non-stop fears of the unknown. It clears my mind for my day. I feel more optimistic, more patient, more loving and surprisingly, more creative. Journalling opened a space within my consciousness that allowed me to witness my thoughts and emotions without letting them define me. Because once they were out of me, I was still there, whole, and complete as the observer.

Emotions and thoughts are transient, ever changing. They provide clues to areas that may need your attention. Writing provides a safe space for you to observe and move through strong emotions, instead of suppressing, ignoring, or taking them out on those around you.

Once you can observe your thoughts and emotions in the physical plane, you immediately open up space inside you that brings you closer to stillness and calm. Your thoughts keep going round and round and often repeat themselves throughout the day. Imagine the act of writing as thoughts coming in and then moving out like clouds passing by in the sky. As you observe and express your thoughts, you will access greater clarity, intuition, and creativity.

From this clear space you make contact with your true Self. When you meet yourself at this level and begin to live more truthfully from your centre, true freedom is possible.

Journal Prompts

1. What do you need to let go of to find more space and stillness in your life? For example, are you over-committed somewhere or are you attached to a belief that's holding you back?

2. What can you add into your daily routine that will bring you a deeper sense of connection with your true Self (e.g., journaling, self-care routine, meditation)?

THE ROLE OF THE EGO

I touched on the ego in Chapter 3 and will elaborate on its role in this section. The ego is so much a part of our daily lives, and we must learn to co-exist with it. The "I" or ego, in this instance, doesn't mean "egotistical" or self-centred. The ego is our sense of self, and it separates us from others. It's our persona that is strengthened by our desires, wants, needs, thoughts, and beliefs about who we are.

It's important to understand that your ego is not bad. In fact, it is the driving force within you that seeks new opportunities, and that yearns to evolve and reach new levels of personal success. The trouble begins when your ego is so strong that it takes over your life and creates continued separateness between yourself and the world around you. Your thoughts pull you out of the present moment and into the uncertain future created in your mind or into the past that you cannot change. The ego is responsible for creating worries and doubts, competition, and comparison rather than collaboration and oneness. It's the voice in your head that never stops thinking until you finally go to sleep.

Your ego is a part of your psyche. When you begin to observe it as such, it will have less control over you. Think of it as that constant voice that tells you what to do all day long. It tells you what to think, how to feel, and how to judge others and yourself. The ego forms opinions of what's good and bad, what's acceptable and not. It directs your entire life, and not always for the good. It also functions best on autopilot—with a learned pattern of beliefs that become easier not to question because they define the "I" that you associate with. It also takes much less cognitive energy to fold into the patterns of the ego. The ego becomes your identity, and it is difficult to question your sense of self. The ego is not always truthful with you. It fools you into thinking you're one way and not another based on learned behaviour patterns from the past.

Think of a time when something happened that forced you to change your plans. It can be a small setback—something that happens daily—or it could be big and life changing. For example, you have a plan to get some work done that you've been procrastinating for a while and the deadline is fast approaching. You get up early, you're ready to start the day, and then the phone rings. Someone or something needs your immediate attention: an emergency equals a setback! The work will not get done as planned.

If you're operating solely from the ego, you may get upset with yourself for the procrastination that led to the present situation. Self-criticism could then kick in and lead to feelings of guilt for not accomplishing what you set out to do. The ego will catch these negative thoughts and take you down a rabbit hole of emotion. The situation is actually neutral. It's your ego that interprets and decides if the external event is going to help or hinder you. It will immediately conjure up a judgment of good or bad, right, or wrong.

The ego reinforces the separation between your sense of "I" and the environment you are interacting with—the people, the situations, the traffic, the weather, the busyness of the grocery store, and everything that is actually happening in the present moment. The events of your day filter down through layers and layers of the self-identity that you have created and solidified over the years. The same situation that causes stress for one person may create relief for another.

The ego continues to gain strength by complaining about people or about situations you find yourself in, or by something that is happening that you believe shouldn't be. The ego may seem like "you" because your sense of self has been reinforced since you were a toddler. Think of the ego as a computer program that's been downloaded into your psyche over the many years you've been on this planet. It's a program that's had upgrades and new versions, but it's fundamentally the same ego: it's just been modified over time.

THE DUALITY OF EGO EMOTIONS

I often imagine a kaleidoscope when I think of the emotional body of the ego. For a very long time and even sometimes now, I thought I had to be one way—that certain emotions were bad and that when I felt anger, sadness, guilt, jealousy, or resentment I was failing in my spiritual journey. I thought the goal of awakening spiritually meant I was supposed to not feel these "bad" emotions so strongly. When I judged and compared myself with others, I later felt shame. When I made decisions based on jealousy, comparison, and judgment, they never felt quite right.

I didn't want to know and feel that shadow part of myself. I wanted to just be joyful and happy. I mean, who willingly wants to look at their dark side? It doesn't really feel that good. I would feel even worse when I judged myself for feeling jealous or angry or resentful. It was like a downward spiral of self-recrimination and making an entire part of myself bad, not good enough, not evolved, and inferior to others.

Looking back with a new perspective, I can see that those feelings provided a starting point that launched me into a period of self-reflection and discovery. Diving into and becoming curious about the human psyche and self-empowerment has directed much of my journey thus far. Here's the liberating truth I've come to understand and embody: the human experience is coloured by every shade of emotion from joy to sadness, love to hurt, acceptance to jealousy, contentment to envy and every shade in between.

It's not all or nothing, black or white, good or bad. There's an array of grey in between and we are never in one shade for too long. An emotional state does not define us. It does not make us who we are. This realization gave me a powerful sense of freedom. It gave me permission to become the observer of the emotion without attaching my true Self to the emotion.

This lesson was further cultivated when I attended a yoga teacher training in 2017. I learned that we have the unique ability to adjust and move through a wide range of emotions. True healing is feeling the not-so-nice emotions, accepting them, and letting them pass through, no matter how long it takes. There is no need to fix, change, hide or feel shame about them. When there is nothing to fix about yourself, you can begin to see yourself as whole and complete exactly as you are. Giving yourself permission to feel without creating more angst and guilt for yourself is where healing begins. Let the adage, "This too shall pass" be your guide. It applies not only to the "bad" feelings, but also the "good" ones. The practice is to accept the present moment no matter what is happening and find the lesson contained within.

Here is an example:

- I know that I am selfish, and I know that I am giving.
- I know that I am free, and I know that I am confined.
- I know that I am loving, and I know that I am angry.
- I know that I am friendly, and I know that I am standoffish.
- I know that I am outgoing, and I know that I am shy.
- I know that I am confident, and I know that I am doubtful.

Doing this exercise can open up a new way of seeing and honouring both the light and shadow aspects of yourself, while knowing neither the light nor dark emotions define who you truly are. There is freedom that comes with complete acceptance of yourself and others exactly as they are. If you feel drained by life, gaining back your vitality can start right here, right now, with acceptance and surrender. You are perfect as you are—all the good, and all the shadows.

REFLECTION

Fill in your own (as many as you want):

I know that I am_____ and I also know that
I am_____.

Don't get caught in identifying with an emotion or trait that you discover. These states are transient and representative of the ego and not your true higher Self.

BREAKING FREE FROM THE EGOS HOLD

You are not your ego. The true essence that is *you* is not your think-ing mind. As we've learned, the ego is only a small part of your psyche, yet it certainly seems to dominate. You have a physical, cognitive, emotional, and spiritual body. All these bodies change over time. Your physical body ages. Your cognitive body adapts the more you interact and learn. Your emotional body shifts from moment to moment as the external environment changes. Your spiritual body awakens as you develop your spiritual practice.

The true Self is buried underneath all of these changing bodies. It's the silent observer that's been with you through all the upgrades and different versions of your ego self, physical self, emotional self, and spiritual self. The true Self goes much deeper and is the only constant in your life. You can start to notice it as the consistent observer of all your thoughts, feelings, emotions, and reactions to external stimuli.

If you can remember all your thoughts, feelings, and emotions from the past year, then you are superhuman. Can you remember what you were thinking about or complaining about on this exact day last year? Likely not. All these parts of you are transient: they flow in and out like clouds. Some are heavier and stick around longer. Some are lighter and move on faster. The goal is not to completely stop your thoughts or feelings because that would be impossible.

The goal is to reduce the time it takes from when you have the thought, notice the pattern, come back to the present and ask yourself (as we learned in Chapter 3), "Is it true?" Is your ego telling you the truth or is it an interpretation from the lens of past experiences? It becomes all too easy to constantly judge our relationships, people's behaviours, our worldviews, and our opinions of how things should be. Are you right? Are others wrong? Maybe, but more accurately, you've simply built a frame of reference around you in order to feel safe and in control. You can give credit to your ego for creating this illusion.

These frames or illusions develop over time and begin in childhood. As we've learned already, young minds are fertile ground for planting ideas. The seeds were planted, and ideas grew. Through your own experiences and circumstances, you have built an identity you refer to as ME. Now you're an adult and with mindful awareness you can start to witness how your thoughts and ideas affect your reality and what you've created. You have a choice every moment to either believe what you've been conditioned to believe about yourself or to challenge your thinking and shift your perspective.

When you begin to question why you believe certain things about yourself and ask yourself if these beliefs are absolutely true, you open yourself up to new possibilities—what Deepak

Chopra calls "pure potentiality." For me, practising meditation has brought freedom. I've learned I have the choice to accept or change what my mind tells me. In this there's so much more peace and acceptance.

Many other thought leaders have used this philosophy to convey that it's not the situation that changes, rather it's what you bring to situations that's important. Your energy, your intentions, and your belief about who you are and what you deserve is what will manifest in your external environment. If you continue to let the old tapes of the ego play on repeat you will continue to get more of what you have right now in this moment.

Look around right now at your family, friends, work situation, health, and well-being. This is the life you've created! Do you like what you see, or do you want something different for your life? If what you see is not what you want, then I invite you to get excited with the fact that you can change it! With some intentional awareness, you can become aware very quickly of the role your thoughts are playing in creating everything about your life as it is right now. To sow the seeds of change is to visualize and feel a new reality. Because what you plant today will play a part in what you create tomorrow.

We come into this world with nothing, and we leave this world with nothing and in between is the glorious experience that we call life.

Get in Touch with your True Self: Breathing Exercise

There's a way out of being held hostage by your ego—stillness

Here is a simple breathing exercise that you can do every day to facilitate a calm, quiet mind and begin to hear the whispers of your true Self. For the next thirty days, commit to starting your day by sitting quietly for five minutes, and then work your way up to ten minutes each day. Sit with your eyes closed and listen to your breathing. Inhale to the count of four and then exhale to the count of six.

Repeat this breath while placing your attention on your heart centre. Pay attention to how you feel in the moment. There is no right or wrong. Even if you think about your day for the entire five minutes, that's okay. When you put your attention on your breath, your thoughts will become quieter. You may notice gaps in your thoughts. It's within these gaps of pure stillness where the busy ego mind lets go and you can start to feel and listen to your truest Self.

Try not to think about or over analyze what occurs during the exercise. Instead, focus on quieting the mind long enough to listen deeply. I have found days when my thoughts will not quiet down, and other days of great clarity and calm. Those are the days when I connect with my knowing and am in the flow. This takes practice, patience, commitment, and trust.

There is a fine balance between the role of the ego and the role of the true Self. Both are equally important. The mindfulness and mediation tools we discussed in Chapters 1 and 2 will help to bring about a deeper sense of ego awareness. As you become more attuned to your thoughts, habits, and beliefs, so too do you become more aware of the deeper presence within you.

Your self-discovery is not an either-or situation, it's a "both–and" situation. The deeper understanding you have of your ego self will lead you to connect with your true Self. This work is necessary if you want to consciously create a life you love in the physical world. Yet, if all of it was stripped away tomorrow, you would still be you. It is my belief that the SOUL that embodies your physical self, never dies. It is eternal. The you without your house, your money, and all your things is still you. It's okay to want, enjoy, and appreciate material things but know that these things do not define your truest, unbounded Self.

REFLECTION

1. Is there an area of your life where the ego is strongest? Look to an area where you feel compelled to complain, compete, compare, or judge.

2. If you broaden your perspective to view the situation from the true Self, where we are all connected, how could the situation change and be more supportive?

PART 2: DISCOVER

"There is no greater gift you can give or receive than to honour your calling. It's why you were born and how you become most truly alive"

— Oprah Winfrey

CHAPTER 5

SIX STEPS TO CREATING AND LIVING A PURPOSE-FILLED LIFE

By now you've had a chance to explore a deeper part of yourself than perhaps you've ever done before. You've become more aware of the voice in your head, your fears (or where you're hiding from your fears), your beliefs, and your thoughts. You've gained a new perspective on the role that obstacles play in your life and why certain patterns keep repeating themselves. You've had a chance to become aware of the stories you've created that either help or hinder how you define yourself. You've also learned some techniques to help you get unstuck from repeating patterns, negative thoughts, and beliefs. This preliminary work has given you the opportunity to explore your inner self on a deeper level.

FROM LEARNING TO ACTION

Now we shift to discovering practical tools to take all that you've learned and put them into actionable steps. For me, deciding to take action means the difference between just taking in new information and using it to make real, lasting changes.

These six steps are the ingredients you need to move your life forward in the direction of your dreams. Like a recipe, they provide a guide or a path to follow. You may add a little more or a little less of an ingredient, but each ingredient is important. In the same way, each of the six steps is an equally important part of the recipe.

Congratulate and acknowledge yourself for making it this far—for doing the work and asking and answering some tough questions. Success is truly an inside job and there is no better way to positively impact the world than starting with yourself. It is virtually impossible to measure the impact your words, your craft, and your work have on others. So, keep going. What follows in this next chapter are the six steps to creating and living a purpose-filled life. These steps will allow you to realize your highest potential and experience true freedom and fulfillment. By the end of Part 2, you will have a clear path so you can begin matching your purpose and desires with your everyday reality.

THE 6 STEPS TO CREATING AND LIVING A PURPOSE-FILLED LIFE

The six steps, described in the next section, are:

1. Discover your core values

2. Find clarity

3. Commit to action

4. Be consistent

5. Offer yourself compassion

6. Build connection and community

Step 1: Discover Your Core Values

You are unique and embracing that uniqueness is what will allow you to not only be successful but to positively impact others around you. Part of what makes you unique are your individual core values. You may not even be aware of them, but they've been guiding your decisions every day, consciously or unconsciously. If you look around at your life right now, your relationships with your family and friends, your work or school life, and the state of your physical and mental well-being, you'll begin to find a common thread weaving throughout.

You'll either love what you see, or you'll see where an adjustment is needed. You will find things you love about your life and discover areas you seek to change. Your core values are always there, though they may shift at various stages in your life with one or two carrying more weight than the others. For example, in my early twenties my education and building my career were more of a priority than starting a family.

Core values are usually formed at key stages in your life where a significant event, either positive or negative, occurred; for example, a big move to a new city, parents divorcing, the birth of a child, the start of a new career, or the death of a loved one. Some events aren't planned, while others you have chosen.

Here's an example from my own life. When I was fourteen, my family moved to a new city. I was in my second term of Grade 9 and was devastated to be leaving behind my friends, my school, and the house I grew up in. At such a pivotal point in my life, everything I knew was changing, and I was worried about losing the friendships I had so valued.

As I started at my new school, I was surprised to find it very easy to make new friends, although I had not thought that this was something I was good at. But because friendship was such a strong core value to me at the time, I made it a priority. I filled my life with people I enjoyed being around and social events. To this day, friendship and connection remain part of my core values. Although family (another core value) has a higher priority for me right now, friendship, connection, and being part of a community continue to be very important.

When you get really clear on what means the most to you, it will get easier and easier to make decisions that are aligned with your core values. Through trial and error, you'll figure out when you've made a decision that goes against your core values and when your decision aligns with these values. You've most likely experienced this many times in your life already.

For example, have you ever decided to do something just to please someone else or because it felt like the popular choice? I know I have. When this happens, you know something feels off. You may experience exhaustion, irritability, stress, or a general feeling of unhappiness. Tasks will feel more difficult, and you may start to blame others for the decision you made that didn't align with you at your core. If you're not centred in your values, this can very easily happen as you get distracted and pulled off course.

On the other hand, when you know your top three core values and use them as a guide to make decisions, not only does the decision-making process get easier, but you're more likely to follow through and be successful. You'll also feel more fulfilled while engaging in the task or activity.

Core Values Exercise

There's a simple exercise you can do to narrow down the hundreds of core values to three or four that resonate most for you. Below is a list of core values that you will use in the following exercise:

1. Begin by choosing ten core values from the list below that really stand out to you as important. Circle them or write them down.

Achievement	Fame	Optimism
Adventure	Family	Peace
Authenticity	Freedom	Pleasure
Authority	Friendships	Poise
Autonomy	Fun	Popularity
Balance	Growth	Recognition
Beauty	Happiness	Religion
Boldness	Honesty	Reputation
Compassion	Humour	Respect
Challenge	Influence	Responsibility
Citizenship	Inner Harmony	Security
Community	Justice	Self-Respect
Competency	Kindness	Service
Connection	Knowledge	Spirituality
Contribution	Leadership	Stability
Creativity	Learning	Success
Curiosity	Love	Status
Determination	Loyalty	Trustworthiness
Fairness	Meaningful Work	Wealth
Faith	Openness	Wisdom

2. Then out of those ten, choose five that currently carry a bit more weight in your life. Some may be similar so you can group them under one stronger value heading.

3. Now out of those five, eliminate two, and choose your final three. It may seem impossible but remember it's not that you no longer appreciate other values, but rather there are three that are most important to you right now. Also know that these levels of importance may shift as you move through various stages of your life.

4. Write down the three most important core values you have right now. Put them on notes in your journal, or on

sticky notes around the house, or even as a screensaver on your phone.

Try to do this exercise every year as your core values may change slightly to mirror your current life circumstances.

My most recent completion of this exercise revealed three core values:

- Freedom
- Connection
- Love

I can now use these core values to decide what actions I will take in the next days, weeks, months, years, and throughout my life that will be the most rewarding and fulfilling. Next, you can turn these values into verbs (actions), and they become the building blocks for creating your life instead of being pulled in and out of circumstances and distractions.

Core values in action:

- Choose freedom
- Make connections
- Cultivate love

Taking this one step further, what do these actions look like in your everyday interactions? What does choosing freedom look like? How do you make connections on a regular basis? What actions cultivate love in your relationships? Once you choose to action these things daily, habits develop and you'll begin to see shifts in your outer world that match your inner desires.

This core values exercise is imperative as we move to the second step: clarity.

Step 2: Find Clarity

"What's achievable isn't always what's important."

— Brendon Burchard

Working to achieve everything will lead to burnout and dissatisfaction. You may have the drive to succeed and the willpower to achieve, yet this could still leave you feeling empty inside. You may be great at checking off to-do lists and accomplishing weekly tasks. There's nothing wrong with this practice. But are you blocking off enough time to add in the things that light you up and are important to you? Are you scheduling in time to rest and recharge? Or are you just left feeling exhausted and unfulfilled at the end of the day? It takes practice and commitment to prioritize the things you love to do. Life can get so overrun with daily tasks that we often forget to sprinkle in the things that bring us joy and happiness.

Brendon Burchard is a high-performance coach and researcher who found that clarity was a key factor not only in performing at high levels, but also in feeling fulfilled. In his book, *"High Performance Habits"*, he writes: "The essential habit of seeking clarity helps keep you engaged, growing and fulfilled in the long haul" (p. 59).

Becoming clear on what's truly important to you will give you the confidence to say yes or no to projects and activities. We are more connected virtually than ever before. We are constantly inundated with ads, social media events, virtual training, and podcasts. How do you weed through them all without feeling completely overwhelmed? You can ask yourself, what's important to you right now at this point in your life.? If something will move you closer to your goals, it's worth investigating it. If it's the right fit, you can then choose to make the time and/or financial commitment to explore it further. However, you may also decide that it doesn't fit right now. If so, keep moving.

I love to learn new things, but it can sometimes be overwhelming to know what to listen to, what to read, which course to take, and so on. This is just the beginning of a new virtual era where our reach can be local or global. If you are chasing down everything, you will burn out. By moving down the path with clarity in the direction of what matters most to you, you will begin to gain energy rather than feel depleted. Clarity coupled with a strong enough intention within will give you the stamina when challenges come up to keep going in the direction of your dreams. If the "why" is strong enough, the "how" will become clear.

Get Clear on Your Why

Any endeavour requires commitment. No doubt challenges will arise. But when your why is strong enough, the challenges you meet won't be strong enough to set you back. Instead, they'll be a learning experience that reinforces your commitment.

About twelve years ago, I expanded my business, which involved putting my personal finances on the line. It was risky, but I felt confident in my decision as I had done a lot of research, my business was making money, and it had been growing consistently. The expansion felt right. I was building a new location to reach more clients geographically. My "why" was clear. I wanted to bring more healthy options to a greater number of people in an area that was rapidly expanding. I signed the lease and began work on the new location.

The timing was not great. The grand opening of the second location was set to be two days after the due date of my second child, but it was in a perfect location, so I took the opportunity. The new store opened as scheduled, and my son was born right as scheduled on his due date! It was a little hectic to say the least.

For the first seven months, I stayed home with my son and relied on staff to work at both store locations.

Having my son during this time was the first challenge. Then three months after the new store opened, my manager of seven years, who I had heavily relied on to run the store while I was off, left to take a new job. That same year, the economy went into a recession. My largest customer shut down for three months and ended up closing one of its locations, resulting in a major reduction in my revenue. The new location was very slow to pick up momentum and grow at the rate I'd forecasted.

My son began teething, and I was not sleeping. It was a hot mess. But my vision was clear. My "north star" was set on ensuring this expansion was a success not only for serving as many clients as possible, but for my own family's well-being. My conviction was strong, so I shifted my business plan to meet the challenges I was faced with.

A new light of clarity came to me one day. To grow further, I had to let go of what was holding me down, which was the older, original location. When I made the decision to close that store, an immediate weight felt lifted off my shoulders. I had to get laser focused on where the growth potential was and let go of what was beginning to hold me down. I needed to prioritize my core values at that time—family-health-success—and make changes based on these priorities.

Being clear about what's most important to you is an absolute game changer as there will be times when the path becomes scary and doubt creeps in. Having doubts and procrastinating is normal, but these are the moments that have the potential to fuel your fire and propel you right back onto your path. When you are aware of when you've veered off your course, procrastinated, or given into your doubts, the faster you'll be able to get back on track. Instead of being pulled down into the spiral of shame and judgment, reset and get clear on your priorities and begin again. Obstacles are simply gentle reminders to come back to your centre.

Be Open to Shifting Your Vision

There may come a time when the path you keep coming back to shifts. What you thought it would look like may change, and the goals and dreams you had six months ago may be different today. If you try to stick with that original path, you may get frustrated by forcing what no longer fits. This is the point I got to with my business. Having two locations no longer worked, yet I was forcing it, creating more stress, and climbing into more and more debt. Once I shifted my original vision and closed my first location, I created space for my core values of family, health, and success to flourish, and the business became profitable. I had more time to spend with my family and my mental health improved.

Every day, you are a new person with new cells, new energy, and new experiences. Over time, the trajectory of your plan will shift. If you can remain open to this shift and operate from the present moment, opportunities will arise that will point you toward the next step. The present moment is where new ideas are generated, where you are completely in tune with what is actually happening. You are not operating from past beliefs or future worries. You are allowing the flow of energy in the present moment to guide you.

REFLECTION

1. What is one thing you wish you had time for that you are not getting to do?

2. Fill in the blank "When I _____, I feel energized and excited."

3. What is one accomplishment you're proud of and why?

4. What activities could you stop doing that no longer bring you joy?

Get clear in all areas of your life.: Finding clarity applies to your relationships, your social network, your career, your community, and your finances.

Step 3: Commit to Action

> *"Nothing happens until something moves."*
>
> —Albert Einstein

Dreams live in our thoughts and imagination; and humans do a lot of thinking. Of all those thoughts, which ones will bring you closer to achieving the life you want? The answer should be clearer now that you've established your core values and have spent time discovering what brings meaning into your life. Once you've narrowed down what's important to you and what excites you, committing to take action is the next step. No one can do this part for you. You can envision the life you want, write down all your ideas, lean on others for support, but until you take action, the dream will continue to live in your imagination.

I've had many ideas that have come and gone. Not every idea is going to be actionable for you. In fact, it may not even be your idea. We often get caught in the comparison game. A friend or colleague achieves something amazing, so you feel like you should be doing something great too-- you're then led down a rabbit hole of trying to create something similar. This has happened to me when a competitor in my industry does something that I admire. They may launch an amazing new product, run a great contest, open new locations, support a charity I love, and the list goes on. There's no shortage of great ideas. But which one's work for your values and goals?

It's easy to compare yourself to others and feel you must keep up. What if you simply acknowledged those ideas and kept steady on your path instead of getting derailed? I call this the shiny nickel syndrome. You're working hard, focused on your business or project or family, when something glimmery catches your attention and immediately you're off chasing someone else's ideas. It may also be related to FOMO: fear of missing out. What if I miss an opportunity or a great deal? What if I fall behind my colleagues and friends in a certain area of my life? When you are steadfast in your commitment, nothing can pull you off course. You become laser focused because you know what matters to you.

Dr. Larry Dossey, a physician and author of *One Mind: How Our Individual Mind Is Part of a Greater Consciousness and Why It Matters*, explains that there is one universal consciousness or one mind, and that we are all connected. Even our thoughts are collective. Although we cannot see it, thoughts are being shared all the time. Of the more than 40,000 thoughts you have every day, many of them don't even originate in you: they're part of the collective consciousness.

It took me a long time to recognize that all thoughts and emotions already exist, and that I needed to begin to filter out the ideas that were not mine for the executing. Once you are clear on your purpose, pathways begin to appear in your awareness, and your only next step is to commit to the ones that lead you closer to fulfillment.

Practically, this means examining the skills you already have, and learning what skills are needed for living the type of life you desire. Perhaps you need to go back to school. Is there any specialized training you'll need to succeed in your chosen field? Would hiring a life coach be helpful to keep you on track and accountable? Is there a support group of like-minded people you can join—perhaps an exercise class, a spiritual or religious group, a community centre, a business group? What skills do you need to succeed at what you love to do? I wanted to share my love of yoga with others, so I committed to yoga teacher training. Then I wanted to further develop my skills, so I took a hands-on assisting course for yoga postures, as well as a yoga anatomy course, and I became a meditation facilitator. Had I not committed to this training, I would still be dreaming of becoming a yoga teacher

Daily Practice

To become great at something takes practice —and, ideally, daily practice. If you want to become a better cook, you can read recipes, but until you take out the cooking tools, buy the ingredients, and create a meal, it will all just be knowledge in your head. Even after I completed my yoga teacher training, I was still afraid to teach. The only way to get better at it was to actually do it and improve as I went along. Six years later, I'm still practising what I've learned, and sometimes I feel like I've taught a great class, and other times I'm not sure how I got through it.

Taking one step every day toward your goals and the skills you want to develop is a way to make your goals manageable without getting too overwhelmed. Visualizing what your life will look like one, two, five, or ten years into the future is a great practice and yet it can also feel too far away and ultimately unachievable. I know I can get caught up in thinking a project is too big or I tell myself I don't know how to do it, which can completely stop me in my tracks. Here's my way around this dream-snatching fear.

Do one thing every single day that takes you one step closer to your goal.

I began journaling every day to get better at writing and expressing myself. Some days I have very little time, but I can still find five minutes. I committed to writing this book five days a week, even if I only wrote one paragraph a day. Taking action is the only way to move through fear and the inner self-critic. Every day I worry that writing is a waste of my time, and that I have many other things I should be doing. Yet I commit to it because it is important to me. Whatever your desire is, commit to taking one small action step each day. This act will keep the spark lit to carry you through challenges, dark times, doubts, and fears. Do it daily, no matter what. Commit to action.

Find Support and Ask for Help

Each day that I sit down to write, I have doubts. And I know that sharing myself on paper or in person makes me vulnerable to other people's judgment and to negative feedback. Filling your life with people who support you in the most loving way is the fuel that keeps your engine going. You can't do all this important work alone. I admit there were times when it felt like I had no support, but I didn't like asking for help. I believed that if I wanted something done properly, I'd have to do it myself.

Having been let down in the past made me strive to be super-independent. My inner voice would tell me, "You can only count on yourself." I've since learned that this attitude was a protective mechanism in response to trauma. Feeling betrayed or disappointed in others eroded my trust in other people. The attachment to this response may have kept me safe when I needed it to, but it began to hold me back from achieving my vision. You can only go so far alone. Collaboration is the key if you want to accomplish great things.

As my business continued to grow, this "I can do it all myself" attitude became mentally and physically exhausting. It wasn't until I began to ask for help clearly and directly that things began to shift. I had to realize that yes, tasks would not get done the way I would have done them, but through collaboration, I learned a new and possibly better way of doing things. By delegating tasks and asking for support, you can free up time to work on new projects.

There comes a time when you must ask for support in order to move forward. That could mean hiring an assistant, a child care-giver, a life coach, or a housecleaner—or asking your partner to take on a household chore you feel overwhelmed with. Maybe you need more emotional support, so you join a club, or community group, a book club, or hiking group. Whatever support you need, seek it, ask for it, and make the adjustments you need that will assist you with creating a life you absolutely love—one that makes you want to jump out of bed in the morning and start creating.

Once you ask for help and people offer you their support, you'll need to take action. When you've committed to others, you're accountable for following through. You can no longer make excuses to cover up the real reasons why you haven't taken the next step. My excuses are usually that I don't have enough time, I don't have enough money, or I don't know how. But I know that those excuses are just a cover up for hidden fears buried just below the surface, so I enter into protection mode. For me, this protection mode is usually a "freeze" response.

I recently completed an advanced yoga teacher training workshop and was asked to implement what I had learned when I taught my next class. I didn't feel ready and was nervous that this new way of teaching was for more "experienced" teachers. So, I put off trying it, not because I didn't know enough or didn't have the time to prepare, but because I was afraid of not getting it right or stumbling on my words.

Then after listening to an inspiring workshop with one of my teachers, I felt the courage to go for it. For support, I invited two fellow teachers to come to the class. I prepared by making notes and following the new outline I had learned, and I mentally set myself up to deliver a great class. I decided to show up, do my best and, above all, believe I had everything I needed to implement the techniques I had learned. The class went really well. I got great feedback from students and from the fellow teachers. Getting through the first class despite my fears developed my confidence and made me realize that the reality was not as awful as I had imagined it would be.

Feel the fear and do it anyway.

You'll likely never be completely free from fear, but you can—with the right support, and with your cheerleaders encouraging you along the way—choose to feel the fear and do it anyway. Notice when you subconsciously block support or make excuses in order to protect yourself from being on the hook. This is the step where you must decide if you're a yes for growth and your vision or if you're committed to playing it small. You always have a choice. What are you a "yes" for?

REFLECTION

1. Is there any specialized training you need to complete as the first step in making your dream a reality?

2. What support do you need to get there? It could be financial or moral support from a friend, a mentor or coach.

3. Who is on your support team? Who would you call on when you want to quit?

4. What is one action you can take today to move away from excuses and be one step closer to living the life you really want?

Step 4: Be Consistent

"Consistency is more important than perfection."

Life is busy and filled with responsibilities. When your days become more about responding to all the distractions, all the to-do lists, all the people who need you now, you begin to get off course. You may not notice it at first, but over time it builds—into resentment, anger, stress, or to always feeling overwhelmed. This further leads to guilt and feeling bad about the things you did not accomplish that were important to you. Have you ever said to yourself, "I would love to _____, but I have so many other things to do. I know I have! There is a way out and you're already halfway there if you've made it this far in the book.

Once you've established what's important to you (core values), you're clear on what you must do (clarity) and you've taken at least one step into creating what's important to you (commitment), the next step is to make it consistent. In the beginning, you may be highly motivated, excited, and energized to get going. The next step is to start practising it consistently, but there will be days when you don't feel like exercising, writing your blog, meditating, doing yoga, contacting possible new clients, or working on your business plan. But if you schedule it into your calendar and develop a consistent routine, your only task is to show up.

Some days you will rock it. You'll be on fire, lit up, motivated, and super-productive. Other times you may show up, write a few words, get stuck, or be forced to take many breaks in your exercise routine. Whatever the activity, know that by showing up daily and consistently while honouring the outcome and how you feel, you'll begin to develop the habits that will take you to the next level of creating your best life.

When you see a wildly successful person, you never see the months, days, and hours it took them to get there. You may look at them with admiration and wonder how they make it look so easy. It's not luck. It's because of a consistent, daily practice of showing up for the hard work even when you don't feel like it—because your why is bigger than that moment's distractions.

Inspired Action

I love the example of exercising because I think most folks have experienced this before. Do you want to feel good, be healthy, and have enough energy to live each day to its fullest—and live a long healthy life? To achieve this, you must commit to a routine of moving your body and nourishing it with healthy food. Yet many people struggle with this. Not having enough time is often a factor. The question is, will you ever have enough time if you don't make healthy habits a priority? If you suddenly had the time, would you do it?

If you're unsure, stand up now and do ten squats. How did it feel? Did you start exercising—yes. Did you do it perfectly? Probably not. But did you start? Yes. You did ten squats. Now what if you committed to doing ten squats every day for thirty days when you brush your teeth? I know that at the end of thirty days your legs will be stronger. If you can give up what it must look like to do it "right," then you are more likely to stick to a routine, thus creating a new healthy habit. It's the story the mind and ego create that complicates simple tasks, not the carrying out of the tasks.

The next sections describe things you can do to move toward inspired action.

Take one small step each day

If you want to achieve any goal, consistent daily practice is the fastest way to get there. What you do today is never a waste of time. Every small step you take will compound and lead you to the next step, and the next.

- If you want to start a business, can you work on a business plan for one hour a day?
- If you want to run five kilometres, can you start by running just one kilometre daily or walk the five kilometres?
- If you want to write a book, can you write for thirty minutes a day?
- If you want to be a speaker, can you practise for ten minutes a day?
- If you want to have a deeper connection with a friend or loved one, can you call them daily to see how they're doing or set up a weekly coffee date?

If the goal is important enough to you, you will find the time. If the excuse of not having enough time is not the true reason, I invite you to look deeper.

Start journaling

It can be helpful to journal on what is holding you back from taking consistent action. The first thing that pops into your head is often what will lead you deeper into the story that continues to have its grip on you. Grab a pen and paper. Don't use a computer or you'll just end up correcting all your typing errors. Set a timer and journal for five minutes without stopping, editing, or fixing. Just write whatever comes to mind and be honest with yourself. This exercise is just for you. You don't have to share it, and in fact you can even rip up what you write into tiny pieces after and destroy it. The point here is to just get it out of your head and onto the paper so you can start to become aware of any blocks that may be holding you back.

Try visualization

Another helpful tool is visualization. Envision how you want to feel six months from now. Imagine who is with you, and what your space looks like. Are you working in an office or outdoors? Are you giving a presentation? Are you teaching your favourite subject? Are you leading a group? Are you in the best shape of your life? Now begin to work backwards. What is one thing you could do every single day to get you closer to this six-month you? Working backwards from the end is a great way to determine how long something will take to complete so you can set realistic goals. You may discover you need more or less time to complete your project or goal than you had anticipated. Developing these smaller milestones will help to keep you inspired and engaged.

This technique can also bring clarity to areas where you may need extra time and support or where you can adjust the plan. For example, in my business I like to develop annual sales targets. I start out with an annual target then I work backwards and break up my goal into smaller achievable practices so I can determine what sales volume I need to achieve each month, then each week, then each day. I make these goals detailed; for example, I need to pitch my product to "X" number of people. I need to sell "X" amount of product A and B to meet my daily target.

Create a visual calendar

Print out a monthly calendar and fill in one thing you'll do each day for the next thirty days. Remember, it can be just five minutes a day if that's all that's realistic for you. The idea is to not create more stress and tension, which could happen if you feel rushed or if you're being interrupted during your scheduled time frame. Communicate your plan with someone else who can hold you accountable. Set boundaries so you won't be interrupted during your work time. This will help you to be more productive and fulfilled during your creative time.

When I started my meditation practice, I would feel stressed and anxious if I missed a day. I was putting so much pressure on myself to stick to a twenty-minute meditation every morning because I felt like that was the only "right" way to do it to get the best result. I knew this was a counterproductive story because I really do love to meditate and by having such a rigid schedule, I was turning it into a chore rather than a joyful activity to do each day. So, I decided to commit to a daily five-minute practice, which meant that I could consistently keep my stress level down without overcommitting my time and then skipping a day. With this consistency, I felt more patient, more clear, and more accomplished in my meditation practice.

Examine and get clear on your purpose

An important part of taking consistent action is to go back to step 2 and get clear on your purpose, or your "why"—the reason you want to accomplish "X" is a major piece of the puzzle you are working so hard to put together. I invite you to continually visit your own why. When your why, or your purpose, is strong enough, you'll make a consistent effort, but you could easily be pulled off track.

To counterbalance this allure, visit your why as often as you need to. Write it on sticky notes to put on your bathroom mirror where you'll see it every day. Revise your why as it becomes clearer to you. Don't get discouraged if you take some time off, whether planned or not. The time away from your daily practice can be just what you need to come back even stronger and more committed to your goal. Anything worth creating takes time and patience.

Give up perfection

Most importantly, give up the need to do things perfectly. Imagine there was no such thing as perfection and that all you had to do was show up and take one step forward each day. Admittedly, I'm a perfectionist. As we learned earlier on, perfection is unattainable. It's a construct of the ego that keeps you stuck. Know that anything you try will be imperfect. You will make mistakes along the way that could cost you time, money, or a bruised ego—maybe all three. But if you decide to always do your best on any given day, then all of these perceived mistakes or failures turn into learning experiences.

Don't let those roadblocks stop you from starting. If you can get into the mindset that you may look silly, make mistakes, or say the wrong thing, then you can release the grip perfection has on you and just begin where you are. Learn and grow amidst the mess of learning and growing. The support and resources are available to you when you decide to pursue the passions that bring joy to you and others.

REFLECTION

1. Insert dream here:
   I want to_____. To achieve that I commit to
   _____for _____ minutes/hours every day.

2. I want to do this because (insert your **WHY**
   here) _____

3. What could get in your way from taking consistent action?

4. What adjustments could you make to get back on track?

Step 5: Offer Yourself Compassion

"If your compassion does not include yourself, it is incomplete."

—Buddha

If compassion is about understanding other people's pain and wanting to mitigate it, then self-compassion is about understanding your own suffering and doing what you can to ease and soothe yourself. Hold on to self-compassion as you find courage to step outside your comfort zone and into unchartered waters. Making mistakes and having setbacks is completely expected when you're on the path of intentional growth and change.

Self-love + Self-care = Self-compassion

The Importance of Self-Care

Ever since I was a child, I've been driven by my goals. I would set my mind to accomplish something and most of the time succeed, even if it meant I struggled. It started with getting good grades in school. This meant often studying and doing homework when my friends were going out. It also meant staying up late and getting up early to complete assignments to perfection. This continued throughout university and into my first career as a business owner. And it worked on the surface. If you were to view my life as an outsider, you would've seen a university graduate successfully building and managing her own business. I was young, and I had a lot of energy, very few other commitments, and I worked very hard. I filled much of my day working.

But this wasn't sustainable. I began to burn out. I began to feel more anxious than relaxed, more reactionary than calm. I would have outbursts of anger and frustration at the smallest things. Ultimately, I didn't like who I was becoming, and I started to realize my tank was running on empty. The problem was, I wasn't stopping to refuel. I was running fast as someone with a Type A personality, which is associated with being fiercely independent and goal driven. Self-care was a concept that used to feel very selfish to me, and sometimes still does. I had a lot of guilt associated with self-care, much like the guilt associated with asking for help.

You can't move your life forward in a healthy, sustainable way without taking care of yourself. I began to take yoga classes—first once a week and then three to four times a week, along with regular exercise at the gym. I began to fall in love with the way it made me feel. I began to crave physical movement and deep rest. Without it, I was not my best self.

Understanding Type A and Type B Personalities

Cardiologists Ray Rosenman and Meyer Friedman, who in the 1950s introduced the concept of Type A and Type B personalities, were interested in how personality might predict heart disease later in life.

They defined Type A individuals as self-critical and competitive, and compelled to work toward goals without always experiencing much joy in the process or in their accomplishments. These people may multitask and get impatient with delays or anything else that interferes with their productivity. They may also overcommit and end up feeling rushed and stressed as they attempt to complete tasks in unrealistic time frames.

People with Type B personalities, by contrast, are more relaxed, laid back, and even tempered. They often go with the flow when changes occur in their environment. They don't worry or stress as much and are highly flexible. And they are often more patient and creative.

Categorizing personality types has become tremendously detailed since the 1950s. Categories can be based on individualized strengths, weaknesses, work ethics, and personal preferences. These behaviour/personality styles are now commonly used in employment settings, career mapping, and personal development training. They can be highly detailed and complex. In this chapter, I will focus only on Type A and Type B personalities.

Understanding your personality type can be an important tool to gauge when you begin to feel excessive in one way or the other on the spectrum. With awareness, you will start to see when re-centring is necessary. For example, I tend to create a huge to-do list in an effort to feel productive. When I take time to relax—reading a book on the back deck, for example—my inner voice tells me that I'm being lazy.

My tendency toward a Type A personality keeps me in the mindset that relaxing is lazy and unproductive. Because of my addiction to filling the time, I schedule too much into my day and then get overwhelmed and frustrated and lash out at others when they get in the way of my schedule. Not much flexibility here.

It can be easy to slip into a mentality that equates productivity with worthiness. For people who lean toward a Type A personality, this can be draining. Self-care becomes even more important during changes, challenges or reaching for your big dreams. Falling victim to self-criticism and frustration when things are not moving fast enough leads to major energetic blocks. You essentially become your own roadblock.

On the flip side, you may tend toward the Type B personality. This may mean that you are easygoing, flexible, and relaxed, but it may also mean that you take longer to complete tasks or—with no clear deadline—abandon them altogether. You may lack clear boundaries, believing that going with the flow will be easier. And you may keep wishing for things you don't have and feel frustrated when you don't achieve what you set out to accomplish. Visualizing, wishing, and thinking about what you want is important, but staying too long in this space will not amount to accomplishing it. You will need to take action.

Finding yourself too far to the right or left on the continuum can cause stress in different ways. Recognize when you are experiencing a higher level of sustained stress. Not only does chronic stress lead to health issues in the short and long term, but it also hinders your flow of creativity and your ability to think critically and solve problems. It's important to practise self-care and have compassion for who you are and what you need.

Understanding the Natural Stress Response

We encounter stressors every day, from getting stuck in traffic to solving problems at work, to rushing to pick up kids from school. When we experience stress, the hypothalamus, a tiny region at the base of the brain, signals your body that a threat has been detected. This prompts the adrenal glands to produce adrenaline and cortisol hormones. These hormones curb functions that are considered non-essential during a fight-or-flight situation; this includes suppressing the digestive and immune systems and the ability to think creatively. Think of stress as a switch that puts your body into survival mode.

Once the threat has passed, hormones return to their resting state. Cortisol and adrenaline drop, and your heart rate and blood pressure return to normal. All other systems resume their natural activities—you are safe.

The challenge with our lifestyle today is that our fight-or-flight response may be turned on constantly. The feeling that you are in constant survival mode is very real for many people. Prolonged activation of the stress response puts you at risk for many long-term health problems. Self-care isn't selfish. It's critical for long healthy living.

I was on a virtual weekend meditation workshop that involved two days of sitting at my computer for five hours at a time. I loved every minute of it and the time flew by. At the end of the weekend, what I really needed was a long, hot bath, and some relaxation, but I ignored my body's intuitive need for self-care. Instead, I did an hour-long, intense power yoga class.

My body did feel pretty good after, but I was drained and for the next two days I felt exhausted, had a foggy brain, and had very sore glutes! I also pulled a muscle in my neck which was painful and forced me to have to modify my work and my yoga practice. The body does not lie—learn to listen to its cues. I choose not to see these after-effects as a setback, but rather as part of an ongoing opportunity to awaken to how my "I'm not good enough unless I exercise" beliefs can continue to rule my life.

Give Yourself A Break

There is no mountain top to reach to take an Instagram selfie with the caption: "Me in 2020: Finally Reaching Enlightenment." There is no grand prize at the end. This is life and it's happening now, not in the future. The true win is experiencing all the small, daily moments of awakening. It's in realizing that these moments all add up to the big moments of the life you are creating.

Self-compassion is at the root of achieving a healthy mind, healthy emotions, and a healthy body. It's a way to move softly and with love through challenges you face. Out of self-compassion comes less judgment, less reactivity, and a greater understanding and compassion for others. If you can bring compassion to yourself, then you can have compassion for others. Judgment separates: compassion brings us together.

"While the motivational power of self-criticism comes from fear of self-punishment, the motivational power of self-compassion comes from the desire to be healthy."

—Kristin Neff

REFLECTION

~

For this next exercise, try not to get pulled into self-judgment. The more you can shine a light on your blind spots, the faster you can spot them in the future. This awareness will allow you to bounce back out of the external chaos of life and continue to honour and love yourself.

1. For the next twenty-four hours, pay attention to when you are judging yourself for taking on too much or not doing enough. What does that little gremlin voice inside you say?

2. Is there a situation or person, or thing that sends you into an, "I'm not good enough" cycle that in turn causes you to ignore your self-care needs?

3. When do you ignore what your body truly needs? What is the result?

4. Write five self-care activities you can turn to when you begin to feel overwhelmed and stressed out or just need a reset.

Step 6: Community and Connection

Community is any social unit where people share things in common, such as customs, values, or identity. The concept of community can be expanded further to include a group of people who care for each other, or who share interests that invoke a sense of belonging. When you are part of a community, you automatically become a contributor to that group. Whether you do it consciously or unconsciously, your actions have an impact on your community. If you take this one step further, who you are to your community, in addition to what you do, is equally, if not more impactful than the daily tasks you perform.

In a recent yoga class, the teacher said, "Look not at *what* you are doing, but *who* you are being." This really stuck with me—so much so that it's posted on the white board in front of me as I write. There will always be things to do, like "the what": the busy work, the mundane work, the exciting adventures, the milestones in your life, the fun times, the times of grief.

During all the moments that add up to your life, can you look back and see who you were being for yourself and for others? What was your impact on your community of friends, family, co-workers, acquaintances and even strangers? What are your values, your virtues, your non-negotiables? Are you a person who can be counted on to help when needed? Are you a good listener? Do you give great advice? Do you bring a sense of calm to stressful situations? Are you energetic and positive? Are you an avid environmentalist encouraging everyone to be more conscious of waste?

The list can go on and on, but the point is that you are an important contributor to your community—big or small, you have an impact. Be clear on the impact you have and the impact you want to have and notice if there is a gap. This gap provides a great place to start interacting more with your community.

The Importance of Connecting with a Community

Community is a source of support

Having a community that you can lean on for support is incredibly valuable. A community you're deeply connected with will be there to hold you accountable to your goals, encouraging and supporting you to fulfill what is most important to you, especially when you get discouraged. Your community can vary: it may be a group of professional speakers, a business group, an association, a religious group, a parenting group, a cycling group, or a running club—the list goes on.

Having a group or a coach, a friend or mentor that you can meet with regularly is key to realizing your dreams and keeping focused on your vision. There will be times when you get distracted and you may commit to things that take a tremendous amount of time, which don't align with your core values nor move you closer to living a fulfilling life.

Distractions are everywhere—social media, TV, movies, the news, other people who will judge your work, disagree with your choices. There will be times of doubt. Having enough strength and courage to stand behind your choices is a muscle you'll have to build. By having a support system to keep you on track, you will be able to come back faster when other tasks or negative self-talk draw you away. Drawing inspiration from others is like refueling your own tank. Accomplishing great things requires great investment, focus and support. Connecting with a community of like-minded people will get you there faster and allow you to sustain your momentum as you forge new connections opening yourself up to new opportunities and growth.

Being part of a community of like-minded people who care about you can make the difference between action and inertia.

Community allows you to give back

"How can you serve people with excellence and make an extraordinary contribution to the world?"

— Brendon Burchard

Your gifts and talents fall short when you keep them all to yourself. The greatest impact is possible only when you're inspired to create and share your unique talents and strengths with your community. Being generous with your thoughts, ideas, and creations can be life changing for others. Giving back deepens your connection with others and improves their well-being and happiness as well as your own.

When I worked for my family's business, we had a slogan up on the wall that read, "How May I Serve?" For years I would read that statement and ponder it. I didn't fully understand it. How may I serve: Who? You? I? Them? It felt grammatically incorrect to me. But as I grew up, I started to see that it was actually very complete. How may I serve . . . period. What did my customer need from me at the time? What did my staff need? What did the community need?

Sometimes I was an ear to listen to someone who was lonely. Other times I would discuss business or health or our product with a customer. It didn't matter *how* I was serving, but *that* I was serving. I was being generous with my time, my listening, my advice, my creating. I was building a community based on how I could serve, not on what was in it for me. When you begin to build a community out of selflessness, sharing your talents and strengths without any expectation in return, you are connecting with your community on a higher level. It becomes more about who you are being than what you are producing.

Different types of products and services are often not that unique, but who you choose to buy from and connect with is. For example, think of a specialty store that you buy from in your area. Is there a particular person you connect with there, or a certain energy you feel when you walk in? Maybe you have a favourite yoga teacher or exercise instructor or coffee barista. What is it about them that you love, and what keeps you going back? You'll most likely find that it's who that person is being that attracts you to the class they teach or the store they run or the products they sell. These are people who serve with excellence and provide an extraordinary experience by sharing their gifts and talents with their community.

Community connection inspires growth and improves well-being

I'm a strong believer in a good routine because I'm more productive when I have a schedule. I have a routine for a few daily tasks I want to accomplish, including exercise, meditating, writing, and family dinners. I have a whole other routine for my daily work schedule. Within the set times, I allow space for exploration, and this is where I look to my community for inspiration. I don't always do the same exercise, the same meditation, the same writing. I get inspired by my community. The interactions I have with my community of fellow writers may change the course of my writing hour.

Each day I tune into an online yoga class, my body moves in a new and challenging way. I get inspired by the teacher. The teacher provides a new opportunity for awareness that I may not have had before the class. When I choose a meditation, the facilitator opens my mind to a new concept and from there I connect with a deeper part of myself. My community, my team at work, and my clients all contribute to my personal growth and inspire me into the next action. I have consciously chosen communities that inspire me to evolve.

Human beings are wired for connection. Without connection and community, we are at a greater risk of anxiety, depression, loneliness, and physical and cognitive decline. Emma Seppälä of the Stanford Center for Compassion and Altruism Research and Education, and author of *The Happiness Track*, explains the benefits of connection: "People who feel more connected to others have lower levels of anxiety and depression. Moreover, studies show they also have higher self-esteem, greater empathy for others, are more trusting and cooperative and, as a consequence, others are more open to trusting and cooperating with them."

When you find a community that you can relate to, where you share beliefs and values and feel a deep sense of belonging, you will begin to discover a deeper sense of power within yourself. Within your community there will be a space for your uniqueness and your own ideas woven from a common thread.

The yoga community I belong to has a common thread of self-development, acceptance, and support. Each member of that community has their own personal goals and definitions of growth. We are all welcome to explore those deeper parts of ourselves within the community and our yoga practice. Within the routine there is flow, creativity, and the opportunity for our own unique expression.

Having a community will inspire you to grow, share ideas, and give and receive feedback while instilling connection that is integral to creating a fulfilling, meaningful life.

REFLECTION

1. What communities do you currently belong to and why?

2. How does being part of this community support you?

3. Are there any new communities that you would like to be a part of and why?

PART 3: TRANSFORM

"When we are no longer able to change a situation, we are challenged to change ourselves"

— Victor Frankl

CHAPTER 6

CREATING INTENTIONAL CHANGE

Becoming more aware of your beliefs and learning about the important ingredients in your recipe, are key components to living a fulfilling, purpose-filled life. It's equally important to foster an environment that supports you in every way possible. There will be a pull to discard the truths you've uncovered in yourself and your life so far—a pull to drop back into your old habits. The pull is strong, convincing, and powerful mostly because it surrounds you every day in the form of news, social media, magazines, commercials, even music. It's the culture you're surrounded by that calls you to "fit in" and go with the norm because it's easier. Creating lasting, intentional change requires you to fill your physical and energetic space with pieces that not only support you but encourage you to keep going.

FROM THINKING TO DOING TO BEING

We looked at thinking—how you and your beliefs and thoughts create your world.

We examined doing—committing to action, finding a community of support, giving back, and taking care of yourself through self-care and compassion.

Now we'll examine being— embodying and ensuring that your daily choices are consistent with the person you want to be, how you want to feel, and the life you want to live.

Your Physical and Energetic Space

A motto I live by is: *What you fill your space with is what will amplify.* This includes people, books, events you attend, what you watch on TV, the news, social media, and your physical space. These factors have a direct impact on your energy, thoughts, and beliefs. Your ability to create happiness in your life, excel in your career, get through obstacles, and ultimately live your best life is either supported or constrained by what and who you choose to interact with each day. Let's dive a little deeper into how these external forces affect you.

People in Your Life

The people you surround yourself with will affect your energy, whether you engage with them or not, and whether you realize it or not. Some people—sometimes called empaths—are more sensitive to the energy of others. Those who are less sensitive, however, are equally impacted by energy. Have you ever felt uplifted and energized just by being in the same room with someone? Have you ever felt worried, anxious, or unsure and then, after having a good conversation with a friend or colleague, felt more at ease?

Sometimes just being around people with high energy for a few minutes can completely improve your mood. Imagine being in a space with someone who is supportive, loving, generous, and optimistic. You automatically feel happier, energized, inspired, and hopeful. These people are your cheerleaders who can inspire you to make positive changes in creating the life you desire. When you continue to fill your life with supportive people, you will be encouraged and inspired to keep growing in the direction of your Soul's calling.

On the flip side, have you ever walked into a room with others and immediately felt tension and negativity? Being around people who are "glass half empty" types or just in a bad mood can bring you down. Spending a lot of time with them can leave you feeling exhausted and drained. Being aware of the relationships in your life that affect you in this way is important.

It may not be possible to completely remove yourself from the relationship, but it is important to create some distance from it. You can do this by minimizing contact and creating physical or emotional separation. You can intentionally send them love while staying at a safe distance. If it's impossible to remove the person from your physical space, protect your energy by imagining a safe bubble around you. Imagine the person's energy literally bouncing off you and having no impact whatsoever. Send them loving thoughts and move on. Resist the temptation to be sucked into drama and negativity.

Learning to regulate the rollercoaster of emotions you may feel from others is important as it's impossible to avoid every negative situation or person. Also keep in mind that everyone you encounter, whether you define them as positive or negative, is there for you to learn and grow from. It's not that we want to "cancel" or avoid difficult people, as I believe evolution occurs when you bump up against challenges which often comes in the form of relationships. But who you decide to spend most of your time with is crucial. The key people in your life who you are the closest to—a spouse, partner, best friend, or colleague—will either support you or create roadblocks that can hinder your progress. Find your tribe and change your vibe.

REFLECTION

1. Who in your life is a positive influence, someone who you just feel good being around?

2. Who in your life drains your energy or pulls you into drama and negativity?

3. What steps can you take to minimize contact with negativity?

4. What support can you put in place to spend more time with people who uplift you?

News, Books, TV, and Movies

News

Access to 24/7 news coverage can be overwhelming. What you choose to read, watch, and engage in can either drain or uplift your energy. I recently gave myself a seven-day news cleanse—no news for one week. I was so tempted to click the news app button on my phone. I was getting so wrapped up and stressed about the recent news that it was pulling me into a dark space and becoming all consuming.

When I grew up, the news was on at 6:00 p.m. and 11:00 p.m. Today we can get news all the time and it can become overwhelming and distracting. Get the information you need that is relevant to you, then turn it off. Then, turn off all the notifications that pop up on your phone all day long. After I did this, I no longer felt like I was missing out on something. If the news is important enough, someone will inform you. Until then, it's not relevant.

Books, TV, and movies

We live in a society where social constructs—what we call culture—become the norm. Culture includes a group's customs, traditions, values, achievements, and social institutions.

Culture exists on a macro level—in the country, state, or province you live in. And it exists on a micro level—within your community, your work environment, and your family circles. Social systems and culture are woven into books, TV shows, and movies. When ideas become normalized, we forget how they may not be acceptable and inclusive. We cease to question or challenge them and just accept them as "the way things are".

A few years ago, I was watching a karate show with my twelve-year-old son that initially seemed to offer positive messages about treating people fairly and with respect. But as the show progressed, the gender stereotypes became so overwhelming that I was compelled to stop the show and explain to my son the gender biases that were being perpetuated. I was truly shocked how such simple dialogue on a family sitcom could reinforce misogyny as a cultural norm. These concepts get absorbed right into the subconscious mind without you even realizing it.

Cultural norms permeate movies, TV shows, and books and can greatly influence what we believe or don't believe about ourselves and the environment we live in—unless we become aware and begin to deconstruct them. Books written many years ago will reflect the culture of the time period. Reading these books from long ago gives you a glimpse into the day-to-day reality of the time-- like when people of colour had to sit at the back of the bus or weren't allowed in certain restaurants. This was emulated in books and TV programs from that period. This thinking is completely absurd and unacceptable in our culture today, but this was the reality at the time. I often wonder what future societies will think of the beliefs we hold as truths today.

Question everything for yourself and make a conscious choice of what to believe rather than accepting what has been fed to you through various media. In other words, allow yourself the gift of critical thinking.

Think of all the ideas that you're exposed to daily through media. Start being selective with what you watch on TV, especially at night right before bed. When you're tired from the day and you're ready to relax, your brain is more susceptible to absorbing information into your subconscious. It then percolates as you sleep, gets more ingrained and reinforces unconscious patterns.

If you are going to watch something before bed, watch a feel-good show or an uplifting movie. I enjoy a good comedy in the evening as laughter releases all the feel-good hormones that can shift you into a better mind space before bed. But even if it's a program with a positive theme, be aware of the subconscious cultural patterns that are being reinforced. Just the simple awareness of them will be enough to diffuse the power they have over you.

REFLECTION

1. Think of the last TV show or movie you watched. What cultural message was being reinforced?

2. How do these messages affect your beliefs about yourself and others?

3. Have these beliefs influenced a decision you recently made?

Social Media

Facebook, Instagram, Twitter, YouTube, and TikTok are all very powerful social media channels. Since the introduction of social media, you have access to continual, moment-to-moment information. Having such quick access allows you to connect with loved ones, share pictures, and learn about events happening in your area and around the world. Through social media, I've discovered and taken some wonderful online training courses that I never would have heard of without these forums. I've met great thought leaders, listened to inspiring podcasts, and learned about books that I may not have found otherwise.

But you need to be aware of how your time can get sucked away as you scroll and scroll. Filtering out what's important to you and what's not, can be helpful. Ask yourself, who am I following? Do their posts lift me up or bring me down? What am I filling my precious time with? Is it comparison, judgment, anger, resentment, or outrage? Or is it humour, connection, love, compassion, joy, and fun?

Also ask yourself what you are posting and why. Is it uplifting and informative or do you just need to vent? I often need to vent, so I've taken my venting off social media and into a journal. It's not good or fair to anyone to dump all your negative energy onto them. It may make you feel good but consider the energy you're sending out and hence, receiving back. Think about why you're posting, and if it can offer something positive to others before you hit send.

Taking a social media detox is one way to become aware of how it can affect your mood and your day. Turn off all notifications. Remember, the social media giants' job is to bring you back to their page when you've been away. You are the product that they sell to advertisers. Without a product, they don't have anything to sell. It's in their best interest to have you coming back *all the time*. And their algorithms remember what drew you back in, so they start to tailor the notifications just for you, making it more likely you'll click that link. If turning off the notifications doesn't work, remove the app from your phone for a day, and then slowly build up to a week. You'll find that space and clarity return as you see how you really want to spend your time. With all the extra time you have, consider what you can do instead.

REFLECTION

1. How much time do you spend on social media each day? If you're not sure, keep track for a week, and then take an average. Many phones can do this for you and provide a report at the end of the week.

2. If you reduced that time by fifty per cent, how much more free time could be available for you to do what you really want?

Physical Space

Look around you right now. What do you see in your physical space? Is it tidy or cluttered? Do you have positive messages around you or beautiful artwork? Are there things you love in your space? Are there things you don't love that remind you of past events or circumstances you'd rather not rehash? Maybe some things hold old memories or energy that no longer serve you. What in your space is bogging you down? Maybe it's time for a fresh coat of paint, a new desk, a new piece of art, or a plant.

Our personal physical space is often a reflection of our inner space. If your space is full and cluttered, are your thoughts full and cluttered, too? If your space is organized, do you think more clearly? If you're feeling overwhelmed, it's helpful to declutter your space.

Surround yourself with beauty and things that inspire and support you. Consider all of your senses when creating your physical space—sight, sound, smell, touch, and taste.

Sight: Vision is one of your strongest senses. What you see in your environment guides you physically and emotionally.

Look around the room you're in. How is the lighting? Is it soft or harsh, too dark, or too bright? What colours do you see? Is there anything in your space that sparks a reaction in you or is just neutral?

Sound: Sound carries vibration and energy. It can be soothing, distracting, uplifting, depressing and even cause feelings of anger and rage. Think of the type of music that is energizing and inspires you to get through something challenging, like a tough workout. Music can also calm you when you're feeling anxious. I'll often play soft music to inspire my creativity, or something upbeat when I feel tired and need some energy.

What sounds do you hear right now? Are there certain types of music you go to when you need a pick me up or to relax?

Smell: Smells often bring up memories and feelings and can remind you of special moments in your life. When I practise yoga at home, I burn grounding incense, like sandalwood and patchouli, that enhances my practice. I also use essential oils to help me focus my mind or calm me down before bed.

What smells do you love and how can smell affect your energy and mood? Are there certain smells that remind you of something or someone that make you feel good?

Touch: As a baby, my daughter was always soothed by the feel of a soft blanket or sheets. Some people are so sensitive to touch that certain clothing can make them feel uncomfortable and irritated. My sister is very comfortable in two-inch heels—me, not so much! Start to pay attention to how things feel around you physically, including the clothes and shoes you wear every day.

Do you have a comfortable chair or blanket? Maybe a favourite pair of sweatpants or shoes? What is your go-to feel-good outfit? Your most comforting couch or room in the house?

Taste: How can taste affect your energy? For me, brushing my teeth and feeling fresh go hand in hand. Maybe for you it's the taste of a certain gum, or a slice of apple pie, or sip of cappuccino that shifts your energy. Notice the effect certain tastes have on your mood and what memories get conjured. Biting into a favourite food can be comforting and boost feel good hormones in your brain, while tasting something bad can make you lose your appetite.

What taste makes you instantly lose your appetite? What's your favourite taste and what memory does it elicit?

Energetic Space

What you fill your physical space with affects your energy. Every component—the relationships you have, the news you watch, the books you read, the music you listen to, and even the food you eat—has a vibrational frequency that affects you on an energetic level that you cannot see. This is called the subtle energy body and it contains your thoughts and emotions as well. This is why sometimes you just "feel" something is right or not right for you.

We call this our sixth sense, or intuition. The more aware you are of how your physical environment affects your energy the more empowered you will be to make choices that support you. You have a greater amount of control over your energetic space than you may realize. Begin by filling your space with things that make you feel good, that enhance your creativity and inspire you, that soothe you after a bad day. As you notice this energetic shift, you are tuning into your own subtle energy body, and with practice you'll begin to develop and trust your intuition. Your intuition then becomes an unbiased companion that you can rely on as you navigate your chosen path.

MOVEMENT AS A CATALYST FOR CHANGE

Science tells us that everything is energy. This book, the pages, the words, the chair you're sitting on—they are all made up of tiny particles that contain atoms and molecules that, when slowed down, appear solid. Your thoughts, emotions, and experiences are all also made up of pure energy, and these energies can become stuck in the body if they aren't allowed to flow in and out fluidly. The human body was designed to be a conduit for energy to flow through freely, and this energy can build up if it isn't released.

In my business, which is primarily customer service, I occasionally have a client who is not pleased with our policy or products or how a situation was handled by a staff member. We can usually resolve the issue and part ways feeling good about the outcome. But sometimes the conflict can escalate without resolution. I really don't enjoy these confrontational situations. My heart rate increases, my voice shakes, I start to perspire, and my rational, thinking brain shuts down.

In one situation, a client started screaming so loudly on the phone that I had to move the phone away from my ear. By the end of the conversation, I was shaky—my nervous system was all charged up. When I arrived home, I knew I needed to release this energy in a safe, productive way or it would remain with me, and I could inadvertently take out my anger on my husband or kids, or even strangers at the grocery store.

So, I changed my clothes, put on my running shoes, grabbed my weights, and joined a one-hour exercise class. Immediately, my mental focus shifted. I poured my excess energy into lifting weights and doing cardio, followed by a releasing stretch at the end. By the end of that hour, relief flooded over me, and I continued with the rest of my evening feeling good. That energy had to be released.

Young children are much more sensitive and open and feel subtle energies. When my children attended preschool, their teachers would often comment on how good they were, how they shared toys and listened well. But often, as soon as we'd get home from preschool and into a more familiar space, the smallest thing would set them off into a full-on tantrum: they had been holding onto so much pent-up energy that they would explode with emotion.

Think about all the stressors in your day. You must be a certain way at school or work, while driving, or hearing bad news. Stressful energy can build up just the same way as it does for a child. You hold onto it and act respectfully because that's what adults do. But if energy is not released in a safe healthy way, it continues to build up and can lead to dis-ease in the body. Additionally, the added stress weakens the immune system, making you more susceptible to colds and flus, so it's essential to incorporate a healthy way to release this energy every day.

Moving your body is a great way to release energy and create a shift. It inspires and creates change both physically and mentally. Movement is an access point to creating lasting change.

Movement can be anything you enjoy doing that shifts the energy in the body: yoga, a walk or run, tai chi and strength training are examples of how you can create an energetic shift. With conscious intention you can begin to transmute a stressful state into a more clear, calm, and energetic state. Being still in meditation is another way to create an energetic shift while giving your physical body a rest. You can even meditate when you're sick. Lie in bed and consciously move your breath in and out with the intention of healing.

When you move with the intention of releasing and revitalizing, you will feel a shift. This shift is the release of energy. Just like water that flows over rocks in a mountain stream and picks up the rocks' minerals along the way, so does your energy field. Imagine you're a magnet, attracting things to you, whether good or bad, because energy has no preference. Releasing this excess is as important as drinking water to flush toxins is. Movement flushes out the stagnant, heavy energy you pick up, just as water cleanses toxins out of our cells and leaves you feeling refreshed and energized.

If you feel stuck or sluggish, sad, or impervious, try ten to twenty minutes a day of gentle yoga flow, weight training, or a grounding walk or run. Even with just ten minutes a day, the shift will be noticeable. Consistency is the key. You do not have to run for an hour. Simply set ten minutes aside every day for your favourite activity and move with the intention of shifting your energy and letting go of energy that is not yours. Moving your body every single day will bring lasting change. It can signal a new way of life—a new lifestyle, and real change.

The Power of Yoga

The practice of yoga has impacted my life and facilitated a great deal of healing for me in so many ways—spiritually, physically, and mentally. I've been on a journey of conscious growth for two decades, searching my soul for deep fulfillment and purpose. It's easy to get derailed or distracted and to accept your habitual, default life even if it's not fulfilling, but rather just good enough. Daily, mindful movement is a gateway to connecting body, mind, and soul.

I was an active child who loved playing sports, biking, running, swimming, and when I got a bit older, I would go to the gym with my dad for a workout. Throughout my teenage and young adult years, I stayed active with cardio classes, weight training, and running. It wasn't until I found yoga that I began to realize that although I'd been physically taking care of my body, I was ignoring my mental and spiritual health. I discovered I was moving my body from a place of not being good enough, thin enough, strong enough. I had to prove my worth by excelling in sports, and when that got harder and more competitive, I quit. I exercised not to feel good inside, but to stay slim and uphold an image of looking good for others.

One day, I was at the grocery shopping when a man stopped to ask me how I stayed in such great shape. I said something like, "Well, I get in my exercise first thing in the morning, so I don't make any excuses during the rest of the day. Consistency is the key!" That sounded true on the surface, but it was a lie, a cover up, a mask. As I walked away, I thought, "I'm motivated to stay in shape because I don't feel good about myself if I don't. I don't want to gain weight and be out of shape. What will people think? Will they treat me differently?"

I realized in that moment that my drive to exercise and stay in shape was motivated by years of body shame. That little interaction was an "aha" moment for me and started me on a quest to discover what movement really meant to me. When I discovered the practice of yoga, I noticed an immediate shift at a deeper level. I continued to get physically stronger, but what truly fascinated me was how my soul finally began to feel nourished, and I felt better on all levels. This transformation did not happen overnight but continues to evolve as my life circumstances change.

In practising yoga, you will get physically stronger, you will tone your muscles, and you will become more flexible. But yoga also helps to interrupt the steady stream of thoughts that play on repeat day after day. If you want to create lasting changes in your life, you have to interrupt the thoughts that are no longer serving you and make a new choice to send them in a new direction.

Yoga challenges you to stay present through movement and breath—to see what's important now. By being in total present moment awareness, you become the observer of repetitive thought patterns and beliefs. When you can look these thoughts and beliefs in the eye, and decide in that moment, to see them for what they are—fleeting conditioned patterns moving in and out of your experiences—you will have taken a huge step towards your own empowerment.

Whether you choose yoga or another form of physical movement, consider that *conscious* movement has the power to clarify and solidify the change you've been looking for. It's the catalyst you've been waiting for. Let physical movement be your first step in the right direction toward the lasting change you've been searching for.

Set Yourself Up for Success

When you first begin something, there's a surge of motivation. You may be inspired by a desire to feel better and get healthy, to improve your energy and mental and physical well-being, or to connect with others with a common interest.

When my kids were little, I used to wake up at 5:30 a.m. to attend a 6:00 a.m. yoga class. This was the only uninterrupted time I had to myself. I'm not a morning person, so it was challenging. But I was motivated to take care of my body and reduce my stress. The 6:00 a.m. practices lasted for about sixty days, and then my drive began to wane. I started sleeping in, skipping classes, and finding excuses not to go to class: the weather was bad, I didn't get enough sleep, or I had plans later that evening, so

I needed to have enough energy for that. There was no shortage of excuses.

The truth is, there will always be an excuse or a valid reason that pulls you off course and *that is okay*. Ask yourself now, when life gets busy or you get sick, how can you maintain your daily movement? At the end of this chapter, I list several things you can do, even when you're pressed for time or feeling under the weather. Listen to your body and take whatever rest you need. Your life is complex and always changing. What fits today may not fit next week or next month, because you are constantly changing, and so is your schedule and your life circumstances. Give yourself a break, take the pressure off, but come back when you're ready. Adapt your routine as much as you need and stick with it.

Ask yourself, can intentional movement naturally become part of your everyday life? A new habit? I'll share with you a typical week for me. Most of the activities I do at home with no exercise equipment. I usually just roll out of bed, brush my teeth, place my yoga mat down, and get started. It's helpful to have a number of activities to choose from to keep you in movement, like a buffet of exercises.

- Monday, 7:00 a.m.—10-minute meditation
- Tuesday, 6:30 a.m.—30-minute yoga flow (online)
- Wednesday: 5:00 p.m.—30-minute walk
  (weather permitting)
- Thursday, 5:00 p.m.—60-minute in-studio hot yoga session
- Friday, 9:00 a.m.—30-minute yoga flow (online)
- Saturday, 9:00 a.m.—10-minute meditation
- Sunday, 11:00 a.m.—60-minutes yoga flow (online)

Three hours and thirty minutes is my typical weekly commitment. You get to choose your time commitment and your activity. It doesn't have to be long. You could start with five minutes of meditation every morning. If morning doesn't work, you can choose another time of day, but as the day progresses, so do distractions.

Try to choose the same time of day each day. This will build consistency and, as you begin to feel the benefits of a movement routine, you'll begin to crave this time to yourself and it will become a habit, just like brushing your teeth or having a morning coffee.

The biggest shift will happen with daily consistent movement and meditation. On the days when your body needs rest, stretch, or do some light yoga. When you need to connect with others, head into a group fitness or yoga class. If you need solitude and grounding, go for a hike, canoe, kayak, or walk. There are countless activities you could do to clear the mental clutter, connect with yourself, stretch your body, and build strength. Below, I've listed a few of my favourites, but feel free to add your own.

It's about starting to pay attention to how you're feeling and then discovering how you can best support yourself. Engaging in activities that keep you moving will also keep you mindful and mentally sharp. Your active mind will become a participant in your growth instead of a hindrance.

Daily Mind and Movement Activities

Mindfulness

Immerse yourself in an activity that brings you joy and calm and requires your complete attention. Some ideas include:

- meditation
- reading
- creating (e.g., painting, drawing, colouring, writing, building models)
- gardening

Body movement

Any type of physical activity that you enjoy such as:

- practising yoga
- walking
- hiking
- skiing
- snowshoeing
- cycling
- dancing
- doing high-impact interval training (HIIT)
- weightlifting
- running

Mental movement

What challenges your brain? What keeps you sharp?

- doing puzzles
- playing board games
- researching a new project
- learning a new skill (e.g., cooking, sewing, fixing a car, woodworking, sign making, glass blowing)

REFLECTION

This daily commitment takes discipline. Ask yourself:

1. What is at stake for me (e.g., your physical health, mental health, relationships)?

2. What happens if nothing changes in my current situation? (In other words, what is my default life?)

3. By implementing daily movement into my life, how can I see myself and my circumstances changing (e.g., better health, happier, less stress, improved relationships, new friendships)?

4. How will it feel to get physically and mentally fit and regularly connect with others?

"Don't wait for everything to be perfect before you decide to enjoy your life."

—Joyce Meyer

CHAPTER 7

THE REAL WIN

RELEASE THE OUTCOME

What if you follow the steps, commit to doing the work, but don't achieve the outcome you were hoping for? This is frustrating. We're raised to believe that if we follow the recipe and do all the right things, then we'll be rewarded by the results we set out to achieve. However, if we don't achieve the desired outcome, it can feel like we failed. Our inner critic will start speaking loudly telling us things like, we're just not the right person for the job, or that our goal was too optimistic, or that we did something wrong.

Imagine trying a new recipe for the first time. You head out to the grocery store, buy all the correct ingredients, follow the steps correctly, and the recipe just doesn't turn out quite right. For me, when that happens, I can only wonder what I did wrong. It may take me another five or six tries, making a few adjustments, before I'm satisfied with the outcome. But, if I don't even try or get discouraged and give up, I'll never discover new meals that I love. And frankly, eating the same meals for the rest of my life feels boring.

Seth Godin writes in his book *The Practice: Shipping Creative Work* that "a good decision does not mean a good outcome. A good decision is based on what we know of the options and the odds. A good outcome happens, or it doesn't" (p. 26). Read that again! I absolutely love this perspective because it takes the pressure off—like a boiling kettle releasing the steam or a big exhale after a tense situation. Can you imagine just for a moment creating something for the pure joy of it, rather than creating for approval, acceptance, fame, or fortune? Outcomes are never guaranteed, but what is guaranteed, if you shift your attention to the present moment, is pure fulfillment, joy, and connection to your work.

Shift your perspective and begin to see that YOUR WORK is your outcome. The act of writing, painting, serving clients, cooking, baking, parenting, or leading is the outcome. Each interaction you have, each conversation, proposal, piece of art, chapter written, cake baked, contains within it a part of yourself. When you're open to shifting your perspective from, "What's in it for me?" to "This is IT for me," you show up to each activity giving your best in that moment. The results will unfold from here as they should for the highest good of all. This perspective requires a level of faith and trust.

Being conscious of your intention and the energy you're bringing, then becomes the most important part of the choices you make and every interaction you have—the energy you bring to a business meeting, the tone of your voice when speaking to your child, and the choice of your words, carry so much power. When the practice of being present and self-aware is your goal, you will always succeed. There are too many variables and random events that happen that you cannot control, so you can't predict an outcome, but self-awareness is something you can achieve.

In 2020, the COVID-19 pandemic affected lives all over the world. Every country and every person was affected in some way. There was no ignoring or hiding from it. No amount of planning could have prepared us for this type of global event. Strong stable businesses closed. Careers and dreams were put on hold. Jobs were lost due to downsizing or closures. Families were torn apart by isolation or illness.

I humbly admit that I'm an over-planner and perfectionist. I thought I had everything figured out at the beginning of 2020. My business was thriving, my team was jiving. I had solid plans for my team and business growth. My life was pretty good, and I was on track to meet my financial goals at the time. Then in March 2020, when the COVID-19 pandemic hit, my best laid plans came to a screeching halt. Panic and fear arose, so I pushed and pushed to predict and plan the outcome I so desperately desired. As the landscape continued to change, my plan adapted, but not with ease, rather with stress and anxiety. I did not trust; I did not have faith. My best guess was that we'd be up and back to normal in a month, two at the most.

Fear of the unknown, and the need to constantly shift my "plan" became so physically and mentally draining during this time. The only choice I was left with—besides continued anxiety attacks—was to begin the work of accepting what was and letting go of my desired outcome. I had to re-learn that choosing growth over comfort was the only way through. I had to lean into my faith and re-discover what brought me joy. I had to ground myself each day in the present moment and choose to do more of the things I loved, just for the pure sake of fulfillment.

I joined a writer's group and began writing every morning before work. I connected with others who had a shared passion for writing. The daily writing slowly transformed into what is now the book you are reading. My intention was to write because I loved it and the energy I showed up with each morning was joy. From the ashes rose a newfound love. Prior to this, producing a book was not even in my realm of possibility. And so, it raises the questions:

"If you are so set in a desired outcome, what are you closing yourself off to?"

"Are you so set in getting what you think you want and need that you put the blinders on to what else is possible for you?"

I promise you that if you begin to live your life from a place of acceptance and joy, you'll see that you already have everything you need. The universe will respond and deliver more than you could ever have imagined.

We could say that the pandemic caused many things to fail but failure is simply a human thought concept. Failure is not even an option when you let go of the desired outcome. All the work you do, all the goals you strive for, all the time and effort you put in cannot only be about the desired outcome. Living a purposeful, fulfilling life will be difficult if you are only happy when you achieve what you set out to do. When you experience external success, of course, acknowledge, and celebrate it. But to find deeper meaning and fulfillment on your journey, you must be in the practice of showing up and doing your best, no matter the outcome.

On the wall of the ashram where Mother Theresa lived is a poem by Kent M. Keith that I love. Here is an excerpt:

Give the world the best you have,
and it may never be enough;
Give them the best you've got anyway.
You see, in the final analysis, it is between you and your God;
it was never between you and them anyway.

TRUE PURPOSE

The most important question now becomes: How can you be a vessel for creativity, generosity, love, comfort, compassion, and service? You were born with a special set of gifts and talents and being able to share those superpowers in your everyday life is a gift.

*When you stop waiting to be the best, or to develop the perfect skill set, then you can begin right now to share the most cherished part of this life with others—**your unique self.***

This is your **true purpose**. This is where your skills, talents, and strengths become your greatest contribution, which then becomes your source of deepest fulfillment. Part of the process of living a fulfilled life is stepping outside your comfort zone. It means quieting the inner voice of doubt and fear that will try its best to protect you from failure. When I hear my inner critic now, I get excited because I know I'm close to taking a step that will lead me beyond what I can see right now. I know I'm onto something that will challenge me to overcome my doubts and help me become more comfortable with uncertainty.

When doubt and fear are present, it can feel like you're stuck in the mud, unable to step in any direction because you feel safe in the centre of the pit. I call this freeze mode. The problem with freeze mode is that it creates a false sense of safety—an illusion. It hinders the natural progression of living your true purpose. By staying in the centre of the pit, it will get harder and harder to step out. You may even begin to sink. The goal then is to take one step at a time out of the mud and into using your unique gifts each day to serve humanity. Give up what that must look like or how much money you will make or how many followers and likes you'll get on social media.

When I started teaching yoga and only three or four people showed up for class, I would feel so disappointed, and I'd take it very personally—like I wasn't a good enough teacher. It feels natural to equate external validation with our worth. But it's so freeing to instead let the experience of joy validate your true purpose. Whether you reach an external goal or not, the bigger lesson here is about reaching the deeper part of yourself where your Soul can shine no matter what.

Society teaches us to keep striving for more—to make more sales, to buy a nicer car, to own a bigger house, to have more friends. Where does the yearning for more stop and the contentment begin? There will always be someone who has more than you and there will always be those with less than you. The comparison game is a game you will always lose.

The real win comes when you can experience deep fulfillment by generously sharing your unique gifts with others while remaining detached from the outcome and the expectations of the ego.

TRUE FREEDOM

You may see now that you've given yourself the impossible task of controlling outcomes— this is completely understandable. Control is a way to manage chaos. Chaos arises when you don't have a clear path, or you can't see a clear solution. When you experience more unpredictability than clarity, it can feel like the situation is out of your control. To remedy this feeling, you go full force into protector mode and begin to compartmentalize the chaos—attempting to control others and, in essence, the outcome. This control may temporarily feel good, like you've won, but remember, it's temporary. As we learned in Chapter 2, attempting to control the uncontrollable only leads to more anxiety.

But there is another perspective to consider. What if you chose to see this chaos as a collection of synchronistic events occurring to highlight what needs attention, love, and healing within you? It is within this chaos that freedom is born—it is here where you can begin to create anew from a space that is truer for you.

Can you see how this perspective can be so much more creative and freeing?

Even amidst all the terrible loss during the pandemic, I truly believe that the earth, and us humans who inhabit it, were forced to slow down, wake up, and become witness to the deep healing we so desperately need. It allowed us the time to shine a light on what needed the most attention within ourselves and our communities at large. Over the last two years, I've witnessed compassion and collaboration. I've watched people come together and help one another. I've seen families appreciate their time together. I've witnessed regular people sacrifice their own freedom for the health and well-being of strangers. And through these sacrifices, pollution decreased, the ozone layer improved, and even animal populations began to thrive once again. There are wins to celebrate amongst the chaos.

There was a time when I felt angry and upset about some decisions our political leaders were making. I was taking things personally, trying to initiate a different outcome. I was attempting to control something that at the time was out of my field of influence. This led to a conversation with a friend, who said, "Laura, when you can start to accept what is happening, you will have all the freedom and peace in the world." But I resisted and thought, "How can I not be upset and try to change situations that feel so wrong to me?"

When decisions made by others don't match up with your belief system, it can be hard to accept them, especially if they affect you personally. The truth is that no matter how upset I became, I could not change the outcome from that state. Taking on this additional stress and pressure was only affecting my own well-being and the people I was complaining to. This chaos I was perceiving provided me the opportunity to pay attention to what needed healing within me- which was to release the anger I was holding onto so deeply.

It's important to recognize, sometimes the things you're most passionate about can be the fuel needed to elicit changes at higher levels of influence and if this is your path, you will know it and act on it. In this situation, it was not my path at the time, and so I chose another way. I chose to commit to my own peace and allow that to effect change on a smaller, more personal scale.

Every triggering event or challenging relationship you have is an invitation to look within. The trouble is that it's easier to numb than it is to pause and look. We numb with work, food, excessive exercise, shopping, alcohol, other drugs, sex—anything we can to not feel hurt and to feel like we're in control of something. These are all temporary fixes to help move us out of experiencing pain and disappointment. There is no shame here, rather, a deeper awareness of how we have learned to cope.

There are parts of our psyche that became our protectors during difficult times. Growth begins once you are aware of the protective parts of yourself. This awareness gives you the opportunity to see the protection for what it is—a beautiful part of you that helped get you to the place you are now. You then can decide if it is still needed or not. See it, acknowledge it, and make a choice. Conscious choice is the catalyst which will move you from chaos to true freedom.

What you are in control of is your reaction and how you choose to navigate the experience. Even when you have this awareness and logic of viewing an experience as an opportunity for growth, it doesn't mean you don't feel the sting of the situation. It can be challenging to let go and trust that what is happening "to us" is for our highest good. It takes courage to trust that whatever is going on in your life is as it should be.

I invite you to consider that things aren't happening to you; rather, everything is happening *for* you.

REFLECTION

1. Where in your life do you put pressure on yourself to succeed at all costs?

2. The fear of letting go is that you will fall, but what if you let go of the things that were holding you down and you soared?

3. If you could remove one thing that is holding you back from taking a step forward, what would it be?

4. Choose one thing that you do for the pure joy of doing it. Now imagine that you feel that way when you do all your other daily activities. What would your day look like? How would you feel? What impact would you then have on the people around you when you're in this joyful state?

THE POWER OF INTENTION

One of my favourite spiritual teachers, Wayne Dyer, would often quote Victor Hugo, who said: "There's nothing more powerful than an idea whose time has come."

When you are truly ready for change, nothing can get in your way. Self-doubt may creep in, and obstacles may show up, but when you are clear and aligned with your greater purpose you will overcome the challenges. Along the way, you may question the steps required to change and not fully understand them: my request to you is to trust that change happens in small steps. It may not happen the way you wanted or thought. It may feel painful or overwhelming, but there is a bigger picture and larger forces at play.

Greater shifts in awareness around issues like gender equality, racism, violence, and workplace harassment have led people to courageously speak out and stand up for what are no longer acceptable practices. When your intention for change comes from a place of love, truth, beauty, and compassion, you will be more impactful and feel more peaceful inside. You choose to be for a cause instead of against a cause. When you are for love, for belonging, for inclusion, then resistance, anger and hate fade and you can move peacefully toward change for the highest good of everyone. Resistance leads to more resistance and from this space, nothing changes.

When you can stay true to your intention and trust the bigger vision you have for your life, you'll be less likely to get caught up with daily struggles. You will be in tune with the lesson of every situation, which will propel you forward towards a more awakened experience and accelerated personal growth.

REFLECTION

1. How could you impact the global community when you achieve your personal desires and goal?

2. What is the intention behind your desires?

FIND EASE IN THE CHALLENGE

I have always set challenges and milestones for myself as a way to grow and expand. But there was a time when I stopped joining challenges altogether. On a conscious level, I knew my threshold was at capacity and that the challenges of navigating the pandemic at the time, were enough. No more meditation challenges, no more physical yoga challenges, no more new courses. I just stopped.

But, as I took a step back to observe, I realized the real reason I was checking out was due to the pressure I had been putting on myself to give 110 per cent and succeed at all costs. I realized that this pressure was actually holding me back from fully participating authentically: the pressure to succeed, to not let others down, to not let myself down and to not allow myself to fail kept me hiding—I was stuck in the hustle of proving and pushing myself, all to be seen and accepted.

There comes a time when the pressure and the demands of life continue to pile up and escaping them or ignoring them is no longer possible. There is nowhere to run, and you must meet them head on with acceptance. In yoga, the longer you hold a pose, generally the more challenging it becomes. There is a moment when you will have to choose between holding the pose and managing some discomfort, or coming out of it. If you can hold the pose—if you can dig deep, breathe through it, and find calm within you—then a breakthrough is possible, not a break "down." It's not the external physical or mental challenge that causes you to retreat, it's your conditioned, self- limiting, internal dialogue that has you running for safety.

Some of our family's best memories are from beach holidays— from the ocean, the sand, and the warmth. On a recent trip to Costa Rica, we spent our entire seven days on the beach surfing the waves. Getting out past the crest of the wave is challenging. You must observe the waves and enter the water at the right time. However, if you stand at a certain spot, the wave will peak and literally knock you over, and possibly take a piece of clothing down in the process! It's an awful feeling—getting scraped and bruised, with water up your nose.

Day after day, we watched people getting pummeled by the waves. The secret to getting past the point of being knocked down is to watch the wave come to its peak and instead of trying to retreat and run away from it, which is a very natural reaction, you duck into and swim through the wave. It feels scary at first—as if by meeting the wave head on you'll get sucked under. But, by stepping forward at the right time, you come out onto the other side, and it's blissful. On the other side of this crashing wave, you can float and relax amidst the smooth rolling waters.

In the same way, you will face challenges—some small and manageable, some overwhelming and scary that will make you want to retreat. Some will be spaced out, giving you a chance to deal with them one at a time. And others may require you to get some support. If you can become more aware of how you typically handle challenges—fight, flight, or freeze—just like diving through the wave, you'll be able to confront a challenge directly, before reaching your breaking point.

With practice, it gets easier to move through challenges with more compassion for yourself and others. While you may still get pummeled occasionally, don't let this stop your forward progress. You can deal in the moment with anything that comes your way. Remember to ask for support when the wave appears too big: the goal is not to drown, but rather to come through on the other side having learned and grown.

REFLECTION

1. Is there a challenge you have been avoiding for fear of taking on too much or not being able to accomplish the task?

2. If you let go of controlling the experience and expectations, how could you view the challenge as a launching point into something amazing?

3. If you turn down the self-limiting inner voice that is holding you back, what could you accomplish this year?

YOU ARE COMPLETE

"Be happy with what you have, while still working for what you want."

—Helen Keller

As I've mentioned, I have a regular meditation practice. I wanted to give myself a routine and a commitment to the practice to find peace of mind. On some occasions it's been blissful, calm, and clear while on other days the rambling thoughts never quiet down and before I know it, the timer goes off and it feels like I just wasted my time. Even in meditation there's a pull to "do it right" and achieve a blissful five, ten, or twenty minutes of peaceful silence. The strong, stubborn voice of the ego has such a tight grip that it keeps you stuck in a never-ending cascade of thoughts that distract you from being fully present in the moment. These thoughts take you away from what is happening and pull you into lamenting about the past or worrying about the future.

As we've learned already, the voice of the ego always wants more. It's never happy. It's always onto the next moment, task, or desire. And although the thoughts feel like they are truly you, they're not. Your true Self, your Soul, is content and complete: it's the stillness behind all the fears, doubts, wants, and desires. The true Self is the patient observer behind your monkey mind of thoughts and is always there when you're ready to return to its quiet, complete space.

As we examined in Chapter 6, we are bombarded daily with stimuli—from the news, the advertisements, TV shows, Facebook, Instagram, TikTok and other social media—that feed our never-ending stream of thoughts. There are so many things to fill up on when you are feeling incomplete, sad, restless, stressed, or bored. Sometimes your thoughts will steer you in a direction that supports your deeper purpose. Yet if you're choosing from a place of lack, the hunger will never be satisfied. Instead, you will keep moving onto the next thing to fill up the void.

For thirty years I've been on a spiritual journey and have been filling myself up on mostly the "good" stuff—yoga teacher training, meditation training, workshops, conferences led by spiritual leaders, and books on self-improvement and spiritual awakening. The biggest lesson I've learned is that I am—and you are—complete. There is nothing that needs to be fixed. I would never undo all the teachings I've absorbed nor chosen a different path. But in all this searching, I've discovered that I was already whole and complete.

No matter how much you search outside of yourself for things to fill you up, your Soul will always be there patiently waiting for you to return. Continue to choose practices with the higher good in mind—like exercise, meditation, tai chi, and self-development training—and reject the practices that lower your vibrational energy—like alcohol and other drugs, smoking, and overstimulation from news and social media. The high-vibrational practices you're drawn to are perfectly paired with your Soul to keep you steady and centred on your path.

Begin to notice the difference between feeding yourself to fill a void versus choosing activities that enhance your vibration and brighten the light that is already shining bright within you. When your intention is placed on igniting this light, you'll begin to see you are complete no matter what. True freedom and empowerment are possible when you finally stop looking outside yourself for validation and you realize, you're already enough exactly as you are.

REFLECTION

1. What area of your life would you say is going well?

2. How can you acknowledge yourself for what you have accomplished so far in your life?

3. Coming from this place of already being complete, what activities would enhance your well-being?

RESILIENCE

"Resilience is a quality that enables us to move forward after we've processed and accepted loss and change."

— Changeboard

Resilience is not something we're born with. Rather, it's a skill set anyone can learn to develop and strengthen. Knowing what tools and techniques are effective in building a resilient mindset can mean the difference between limiting your potential versus seeing the opportunity in life's uncertainties.

Has anyone ever said to you, "Oh, just get over it"? Or, have you said that to yourself? Why is it so hard to "get over" certain events in our life and move on? Our brains are hard-wired to survive. To do so, they remember the events that negatively impacted us and threatened our survival. This ability to remember is a primitive safety mechanism to literally keep us alive. These stored memories affect the amygdala, which is a tiny part of our brain responsible for how we respond to fear and trauma. When we continue to respond to similar situations from this place of fear, we tend to continue with the downward spiral of negative thinking, thereby perpetuating the less desirable experience.

From this fear-based mindset, we end up making decisions from this same emotional place. In their book *Bounce Forward: The Extraordinary Resilience of Nurse Leadership*, Elle Allison-Napolitano, and Daniel Pesut, write, "We are wired to react and act out habits and emotional patterns that may or may not be useful, but that fit like a comfortable pair of shoes."

During times of immense change, it's useful to remember that we may be reacting out of past habitual patterns of fear to protect ourselves from hurt or danger. It's helpful to remain hyperaware of when the amygdala has taken over our reactions. We build resilience when we can process these emotions without being taken down by them.

Acceptance does not happen overnight, and it may require you to continually check in with yourself so that during times of change or struggle you can move more swiftly through survival mode to thriving mode. The more you practise pausing before reacting to a challenge or triggering situation, the faster you will be able to process changes. As the Bounce Back Project explains, you'll ultimately end up making decisions that are in line with the circumstances of the present moment. This will allow for new possible outcomes and solutions.

Five Practices for Building Resilience

The Bounce Back Project describes five things we can do to become more resilient. They include, self-awareness, mindfulness, self-care, positive relationships, and purpose.

Self-Awareness

This book has been based on getting to know yourself deeply to intentionally create a purpose-filled life. Resilience is built on the same premise. It starts with paying close attention to your internal voice and the dialogue that occurs when something happens that you did not want or expect and had no control over. Developing this skill requires you to be willing and open to examine the way you think about yourself and the world around you, your mental habits, and instinctive responses to negative situations. When something bad happens, rather than jumping into reaction, you can pause, create some distance from the emotional response, and begin to reframe the experience. The more you practise self-awareness with compassion for yourself, the more of a habit it becomes.

"Strength isn't always about being the best, the brightest or the toughest, it's about learning and recovering without ignoring the ways in which your situation has changed."

—Changeboard

Mindfulness

We've already seen how the act of being mindful is an important tool in getting beyond the habitual thought patterns of the mind. Here, again, mindfulness arises as a way to help strengthen your resilience. It involves getting in touch with the observer of your thoughts, feelings, and emotions and becoming hyperaware of the present moment. Mindfulness differs from self-awareness in that it involves paying close attention to your physical actions. This allows you to practice being an unbiased observer, so you can look at a situation without judgment. What makes a situation good or bad is your interpretation of it. By practising mindfulness, you can detach from the reactive, protective part of you and move into the next right action. In stressful experiences, mindfulness gives you the opportunity to build the muscle of resiliency. You learn that you have the ability to handle any situation that is occurring in your life.

Self-Care

With the world constantly throwing challenges at us, it can be easy to feel worn out or unmotivated. Self-care is crucial to maintain and build inner strength. To rebuild your energy and vitality, you need to take time for yourself and engage in activities you love that aren't necessarily attached to a goal or outcome. As I discussed in Chapter 5, notice what activities leave you feeling refreshed and energized. Then start to schedule that time into your daily or weekly calendar. If you typically fill up your days with things to do, try scheduling thirty minutes to one hour a day with nothing on your agenda—just free time. You can then choose to do whatever you enjoy in that time period. This needs to be guilt- free "you" time. If you attach guilt to your self-care practice, you will defeat the purpose of self-care.

Positive Relationships

Having people in your life who you can call on for support will be extremely helpful when you feel overburdened. I thought for a long time that I had to do life alone—that the only person I could count on was myself and to ask for support was weak. It turns out I was dead wrong. Asking for help and surrounding yourself with people who have your back is the only way to flourish. Let others support you, and when they need it, support them too. Connecting with others is part of human nature: it's in our make up. When we're feeling down a supportive friend can be just what we need to keep building the muscle of resilience.

Purpose

Being driven by something outside of yourself can inspire you to remain focused on the bigger picture. You affect and influence others every day, usually by default. Imagine being so intentional and inspired every day that your impact leaves others in their greatness. Fulfilling your purpose brings meaning to you and those around you. Whether you volunteer at a local charity, run a business, are raising children, are part of the church council, coach your kids' soccer team, care for aging parents, or share your knowledge with others in some way, your purpose is present and impactful.

You just have to look right in front of you to see your purpose and impact. Once you start looking, you'll realize just how important your life is. Big or small, reaching thousands of people or reaching one person, everyone has a purpose. Begin to notice yours. Maybe you've been holding back from sharing yourself, your insights, your experiences, and just by looking, just by noticing, your purpose will start to grow and flourish all by itself. This awareness is crucial in building your resilience mindset.

The spiritual teacher and mystic Patanjali said:

> *"When you are inspired by some great purpose, some extraordinary project, all your thoughts break their bonds; your mind transcends limitations, your consciousness expands in every direction, and you find yourself in a new, great, and wonderful world. Dormant forces, faculties, and talents become alive, and you discover yourself to be a greater person by far than you ever dreamed yourself to be."*

The strength to get back up and keep going when you've been knocked down or when you come up against obstacles is found in resilience. Being resilient doesn't mean being static and unbending. To be resilient, you need to be flexible and supple. There is no question whether change is coming, rather, *when* change is change coming. No matter what adversity you are facing, there is always a way to stay focused, motivated, and find a new direction when external circumstances change.

A few years ago, I had a conversation with a teacher I admire. I was explaining to her how I respected her confidence, her openness, and her ability to be so present with me in our conversations. She replied, "What you see and love about me, you already have in yourself. You just need to recognize it, nurture it, and trust it."

Our conversation has stuck with me. Noticing what you love about others is already in you. There is a part of you that may have been buried or that you may not recognize or believe in. Resilience is one of those tools that you've been cultivating since you were able to consciously think. What's usually missing is the belief and the awareness. When I began to look back on my experiences from running my business, I started to notice how resilient I actually was. Yet up until recently, I never believed it. I would admire this quality in others, praise them for it, and wish I could be like them.

I've been fortunate this year, during the pandemic, to witness first-hand the resilience of so many respected business owners, students (including my own children), other parents, teachers, and frontline workers. As a witness, a doorway opens, and you can begin to see the resilience in yourself—to see past the doubt and fear to the powerful impact you have on others when you practice and share your resilience.

REFLECTION

1. Think back to a time in your life when you felt you were resilient. What qualities or values were present for you at that time?

2. Think back to a time when you felt completely defeated and seriously considered giving up. What values and qualities were missing for you then?

3. Is there someone you find resilient who you can connect with or even just think about when you need a boost of confidence to keep going on your path?

FINAL THOUGHTS

You are the creator of your world, the dreamer of your dream. Whether consciously or unconsciously, you are creating all day long. Taking the time to get clear on what your ideal life would look like is an important step to moving closer to it. A great place to start is to notice where there is disharmony in your life. It takes focus, energy, and the right mindset to even begin to look—but it also takes the same amount of energy to stay exactly where you are.

You get to choose. Every single moment of every day, you have a choice. You choose your actions, you choose your thoughts, you choose to stay stuck or to take a step forward. Desire for a more fulfilling, joyful life is not selfish. When you can begin to look at the bigger picture of your impact on those around you when you are in a state of fulfillment, you will see it's not selfish at all; it actually deepens the positive impact you have on those around you.

In the final months of completing this book I was ready to give it all up more than once. I was full of self-doubt and felt unworthy and not good enough to put my work out into the world. My inner critic would say, "There are so many authors who are better than you, who have websites, a literary agent, a publisher, a journalism degree, the expertise" and the list goes on and on. But here's the truth, all of it, and I mean *all of it*, is a story. It's a construct of my belief system that has been reinforced each day by my thoughts, beliefs, and the society I live in.

My request of you, beautiful soul, is to do whatever it takes to live your most fulfilling life. Throw out the rules—they're all just made up anyway. Look past the social constructs telling you what you should and shouldn't be doing to succeed. Instead, focus on doing the things that inspire you and light you up inside, then take aligned action daily. Let go of fixed outcomes. Stay in the ever-changing flow of life and you will be guided to your purpose. Then use your flame of inspiration to light the next candle—becoming the source of light the inspires others to see theirs.

ACKNOWLEDGEMENTS

I have so many people to thank who inspired and supported me in the creation of this book. It was a three year writing journey that would not have been completed without the support of friends, family, and my teachers.

First, I'd like to acknowledge my husband Chris and my children, Sidney and Logan, for allowing me space and time to complete this project. By taking the children away for weekends so I could deep dive into editing without distraction, Chris supported me every step of the way to help bring my dream to reality.

My deepest thanks to Corinne Schroeder, my dear friend, who so graciously offered to read my first, unedited, very messy first draft. My soul sister, Danielle Nimeth, read each chapter in detail making suggestions, comments and keeping my spirits high with her positive re-enforcement. Thank you to Sarah McVanel who created and organized the online writers' group I was a part of 5 days a week for many months during the COVID-19 pandemic. This group held me accountable to show up and write every day and provided valuable resources on how to write and publish a book. Thank you, Diana Ballon, my first-round editor who finessed my words and offered clarity to my concepts.

And finally, thank you to the yoga communities that I've had the honour of being a part of. The teachers I worked with and the students I had the pleasure of teaching provided me with a beautiful source of inspiration and encouragement.

With deepest gratitude and love,
Laura

REFERENCES

- Allison-Napolitano, E. & Pesut, D. (2015). *Bounce Forward: The Extraordinary Resilience of Nurse Leadership.* Silver Spring, MD: American Nurses Association.

- Baron-Reid, C. (2015). *Wisdom of the Oracle: Divination Cards Guidebook.* Carlsbad, CA: Hay House.

- Bounce Back Project. (n.d.). "5 Pillars of Resilience.", accessed March 5, 2022, https://www.feelinggoodmn.org/what-we-do/bounce-back-project-/5-pillars-of-resilience/

- Burchard, B. (2017). *High Performance Habits: How Extraordinary People Become That Way.* Carlsbad, CAL Hay House.

- Changeboard. "What is Resilience?", accessed March 5, 2022 www.changeboard.com/article-details/16347/what-is-resilience-/#:~:text=Resilience%20is%20a%20special%20skill,to%20something%20bad%20or%20unwanted

- Dossey, L. (2013). One Mind: *How Our Individual Mind Is Part of a Greater Consciousness and Why It Matters.* Carlsbad, CA: Hay House.

- Godin, S. (2020). *The Practice: Shipping Creative Work.* New York, NY: Portfolio/Penguin.

- Hay, L. L. (1984). *You Can Heal Your Life.* Carlsbad, CA: Hay House.

- Jain, S. (2021). *Healing Ourselves: Biofield Science and the Future of Health.* Boulder, CO: Sounds True.

- Lipton, B. H. (2016). *The Biology of Belief: Unleashing the Power of Consciousness, Matter & Miracles* (10th anniversary ed.). Carlsbad, CA: Hay House.

- Neff, K., "The Motivational Power of Self-Compassion.," [blog post], accessed November 12, 2021. https://self-compassion.org/the-motivational-power-of-self-compassion

- NeuroHealth Associates. (n.d.). Definitions., accessed September 22, 2021, https://nhahealth.com/brainwaves-the-language/

- Newton, R. (2018), "The Psychology of Conformity or Why do we have the need to fit in?", [blog post], accessed June 20, 2021, www.learning-mind.com/psychology-of-conformity

- Richardson, C. (2019). *The Art of Extreme Self-Care*. Carlsbad, CA: Hay House.

- Ruiz, D. M. (2004). *The Voice of Knowledge: A Practical Guide to Inner Peace*. San Francisco, CA: Amber-Allen Publishing.

- *Science Connected Magazine*. (2018). How Habits are Formed, accessed January 12, 2021, https://magazine.scienceconnected.org/2018/09/how-habits-are-formed/

- Seppälä, E. (2016). *The Happiness Track: How to Apply the Science of Happiness to Accelerate Your Success*. New York: HarperCollins.